DK American College
of Physicians

HOME MEDICAL GUIDE *to*

CORONARY
ARTERY DISEASE

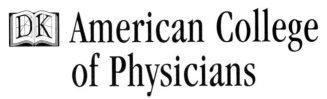

American College of Physicians

HOME MEDICAL GUIDE *to*

CORONARY
ARTERY DISEASE

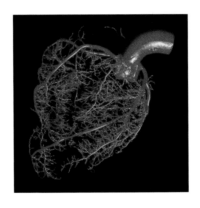

MEDICAL EDITOR
DAVID R. GOLDMANN, MD
ASSOCIATE MEDICAL EDITOR
DAVID A. HOROWITZ, MD

A DORLING KINDERSLEY BOOK

IMPORTANT

The American College of
Physicians (ACP) Home Medical
Guides provide general
information on a wide range of
health and medical topics. These
books are not substitutes for
medical diagnosis, and you should
always consult your doctor on
personal health matters before
undertaking any program of
therapy or treatment. Various
medical organizations have
different guidelines for diagnosis
and treatment of the same
conditions; the American College
of Physicians–American Society of
Internal Medicine (ACP–ASIM)
has tried to present a reasonable
consensus of these opinions.

Material in this book was
reviewed by the ACP–ASIM for
general medical accuracy and
applicability in the United States;
however, the information provided
herein does not necessarily reflect
the specific recommendations
or opinions of the ACP–ASIM.
The naming of any organization,
product, or alternative therapy in
these books is not an ACP–ASIM
endorsement, and the omission of
any such name does not indicate
ACP–ASIM disapproval.

DORLING KINDERSLEY
LONDON, NEW YORK, AUCKLAND, DELHI,
JOHANNESBURG, MUNICH, PARIS, AND SYDNEY

DK www.dk.com

Senior Editors Jill Hamilton, Nicki Lampon
Senior Designer Jan English
DTP Design Jason Little
Editor Nicholas Mulcahy
Medical Consultant Frank E. Silvestry, MD

Senior Managing Editor Martyn Page
Senior Managing Art Editor Bryn Walls

Published in the United States in 2000 by
Dorling Kindersley Publishing, Inc.
95 Madison Avenue, New York, New York 10016

2 4 6 8 10 9 7 5 3 1

Based on an original work by Dr. Christopher Davidson

Library of Congress Catalog Card Number 99-76859
ISBN 0-7894-5154-9

Reproduced by Colourscan, Singapore
Printed and bound in the United States by Quebecor World, Taunton, Massachusetts

Contents

Introduction

This book is about coronary artery disease, or CAD. The coronary arteries are the blood vessels that supply the heart muscle with the oxygen and nutrients that it needs to work properly and remain healthy.

Disease in the coronary arteries builds up over many years and can lead to angina, heart attacks, and sudden death. Over one million Americans a year die from cardiovascular disease, about half of them due to coronary artery disease. Most people know someone who has had a heart attack, often without warning. However, coronary artery disease has not always been as widespread but has become much more common over the last 50 years. We know some of the important factors responsible for this increase.

This book was written to tell you more about this condition, what to do if you have coronary artery disease, and what you can do to prevent it.

There are several terms that are used to describe coronary disease and its effects on the heart. Coronary artery disease is the term used throughout this book, but others used by doctors are explained on page 8.

Coronary artery disease can cause a range of different problems, all resulting from insufficient oxygen reaching the heart muscle. The most common of these problems are:

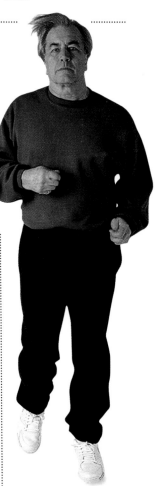

A HEALTHY HEART
Lifestyle factors such as exercise have an important effect on the heart. Regular aerobic exercise will help keep your heart healthy.

Terms that Describe Heart Disease

Doctors use a variety of terms to describe heart disease caused by narrowing of the coronary arteries. The term coronary artery disease (CAD) covers all of these.

CORONARY ARTERY DISEASE (CAD)	Disease of the coronary arteries themselves.
ISCHEMIC HEART DISEASE (IHD)	Narrowing of the blood vessels, resulting in ischemia, or lack of blood supply to the heart muscle.
MYOCARDIAL INFARCTION (MI); CORONARY; CORONARY THROMBOSIS; HEART ATTACK	Death of heart muscle as a result of a blockage in the blood supply.

● **Angina** Chest pain when exercising. Angina can occur during everyday physical effort, not just activities such as aerobics or jogging. The pain decreases when you rest.

● **Heart attack or myocardial infarction (MI)** Severe chest pain resulting from death of an area of heart muscle when the blood supply is cut off completely.

Other conditions that often result from CAD include:

● **Heart failure** Shortness of breath and swollen ankles that result when the heart cannot pump well enough to keep up with the body's demands.

● **Irregularities of heart rhythm (arrhythmias)** Irregular heartbeats that can cause palpitations and shortness of breath.

CAD is not the only disease affecting the heart, but it is by far the most common in western countries. Other heart problems include:

- **Congenital heart disease** Abnormalities of the heart that are present at birth, such as a hole in the heart.
- **Cardiomyopathies** Diseases that primarily affect the heart muscle rather than the arteries.
- **Valvular heart disease** Damage to or abnormalities of any of the four valves that control blood flow within the heart.

WHO GETS HEART DISEASE?

The number of people who get coronary artery disease varies enormously from one country to another and is especially high in developed countries. In general, CAD is a disease of affluence. It is rare in the tropics and developing countries and is most common in North America, northern Europe, Asia, and Australia. It seems to be related to lifestyle because, when people move from the developing countries to a more affluent culture, many more get CAD than those who remained at home. For example, immigrants from Japan who move to the US are even more likely to develop CAD than people who were born in the US.

Within Europe, there are major differences between countries and even between regions within one country. CAD is generally much less common in southern Europe than in the United Kingdom and Scandinavia. This is one of the reasons for the popularity of the Mediterranean diet. Many people believe that eating lots of fresh vegetables, salad, fruit, and fish, and relatively little red meat or dairy products, can help protect against heart disease (see Improving the diet, pp.85–86).

CAD Mortality Rate in the World

Coronary artery disease is generally higher in the more affluent countries than in the developing nations. The mortality rates from CAD are shown for a selection of countries. The rates are particularly high in the former Eastern bloc nations.

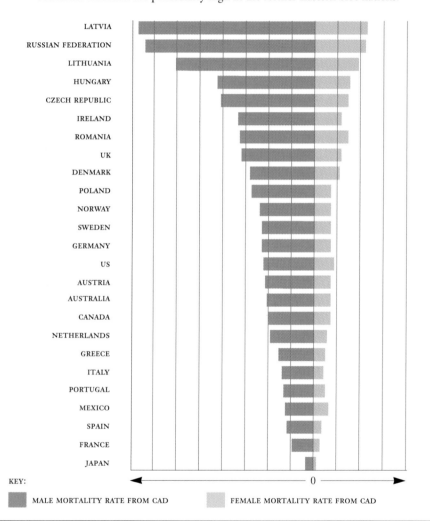

KEY:

0

■ MALE MORTALITY RATE FROM CAD   ■ FEMALE MORTALITY RATE FROM CAD

Although there are descriptions of coronary artery disease that date back to the classical world, it was not recognized to be a common disease until after World War II. Since then, the rates, particularly among young men, have risen alarmingly. In the United States, this number peaked in 1970 but has been falling steadily ever since.

The same decrease has been seen in Australia, New Zealand, and the United Kingdom. Unfortunately, the rates of coronary artery disease are actually now increasing rapidly in European countries in the former Eastern bloc countries, such as Russia and the Baltic states.

It is no exaggeration to say that most hospital beds in the US are occupied by people whose illness is in some way related to hardening of the arteries, and the most common of these illnesses is coronary artery disease. Approximately 7 million Americans have been diagnosed as having CAD. Coronary artery disease is more common than all forms of cancer combined. It is more common in elderly people and four times more common in men than in women until old age. As a cause of death in young men, it is second only to accidents.

Why is CAD so common in the western world? No one knows for sure, but diet, smoking, lack of exercise, and social problems all seem to be likely culprits. Each of these risk factors will be covered in greater detail later in the book.

CAD AND DIET
A healthy diet that includes plenty of fresh vegetables and salad and is low in meat and dairy products helps protect against heart disease.

NEW TREATMENTS

The last 10 years have seen enormous advances in the treatment of CAD. There are new drugs, such as the clot-dissolving medicines that are used during a heart attack, better drugs for angina, and powerful cholesterol-lowering drugs. We have also come to understand the value of some of the older drugs, such as beta blockers and aspirin. Some of these drugs can help relieve symptoms such as pain, and others slow down or even reverse some of the changes caused by the disease.

The biggest advances, however, have been in the use of surgery and angioplasty. Bypass surgery, or coronary artery bypass graft (CABG, often pronounced "cabbage") can transform the life of an angina sufferer and in some cases also reduces the risk of further heart attacks and death. Angioplasty, a technique in which tiny balloons are used to stretch narrowed or blocked arteries, can be very effective, especially now that fine wire mesh stents, or internal supports, are used to keep the arteries open.

This is all good news for anyone who has heart trouble. However, the priority of future medical research should be to tackle the underlying reasons why CAD is so common and to try to prevent it.

KEY POINTS

- CAD is one of the the most common causes of death in North America and western Europe.
- There has been an epidemic of CAD in the twentieth century, which is now declining in the US but rising in countries in eastern Europe.
- New treatments, including bypass surgery, have helped considerably, but prevention remains more effective than cure.

What goes wrong?

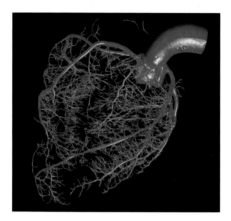

The heart is a muscular pump in the chest that is continually working, pumping blood around your body. It contracts and relaxes 100,000 times a day, and all of this work requires adequate blood supply, which is provided by the coronary arteries.

CORONARY ARTERIES
This resin cast shows the system of arteries that brings blood to the heart. They supply the heart muscles with vital oxygenated blood.

HOW THE HEART WORKS

The basic function of the heart is to pump red blood rich in oxygen and nutrients through large arteries to the rest of the body. When the oxygen has been extracted by the tissues, veins carry the blood, now bluish and low in oxygen, back to the heart.

The heart has two sides, each of which acts as a separate pump. Each of these is subdivided into two chambers, making four chambers in all. The upper two, the atria, act as collecting reservoirs, and the lower ones, the ventricles, contract to pump the blood out of the heart. The right side of the heart receives blood through veins coming from all over the body and pumps blood through the lungs so that it can pick up oxygen. The left side of the heart collects blood that is returning from the lungs and pumps it around the body to the tissues.

The Internal Structure of the Heart

This diagram shows the two pairs of chambers, the left atrium and ventricle and the right atrium and ventricle. Each pair acts as a separate pump. A valve at the exit of each chamber prevents blood from flowing back in the wrong direction.

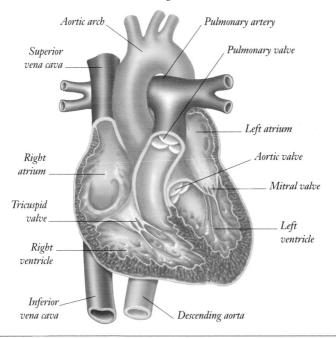

Aortic arch

Pulmonary artery

Superior vena cava

Pulmonary valve

Left atrium

Right atrium

Aortic valve

Mitral valve

Tricuspid valve

Left ventricle

Right ventricle

Inferior vena cava

Descending aorta

In order to reach all of the different organs and muscles throughout the body, blood has to be pumped out of the heart at high pressure. For the heart to act as a pump, the muscle must be very strong and, unlike the muscles in our legs, the heart muscle does not become fatigued. To perform this function, the heart muscle requires a good blood supply, which is provided by the coronary arteries and their branches.

How Blood Circulates Around the Body

Deoxygenated blood from the body organs and tissues enters the right side of the heart and is pumped to the lungs, where it takes up oxygen. Entering the left side of the heart, the oxygenated blood is then pumped to all parts of the body.

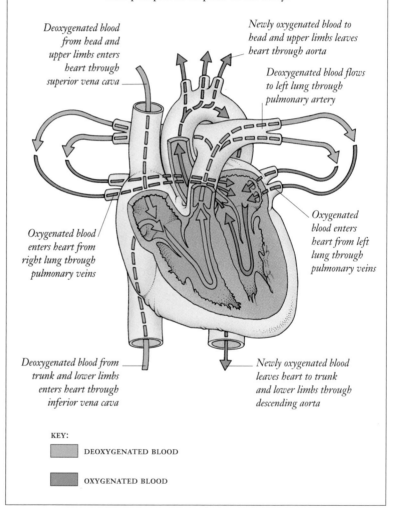

Deoxygenated blood from head and upper limbs enters heart through superior vena cava

Newly oxygenated blood to head and upper limbs leaves heart through aorta

Deoxygenated blood flows to left lung through pulmonary artery

Oxygenated blood enters heart from right lung through pulmonary veins

Oxygenated blood enters heart from left lung through pulmonary veins

Deoxygenated blood from trunk and lower limbs enters heart through inferior vena cava

Newly oxygenated blood leaves heart to trunk and lower limbs through descending aorta

KEY:

☐ DEOXYGENATED BLOOD

☐ OXYGENATED BLOOD

THE CORONARY ARTERIES

The coronary arteries come off the aorta, the main blood vessel from the heart. They are the first arteries to receive blood rich in oxygen from the left ventricle. The two coronary arteries, the right and the left, are relatively small, each about ⅛ inch (3–4 mm) in diameter.

The coronary arteries pass over the surface of the heart, meeting each other at the back and almost forming a circle. When this pattern of blood vessels was first seen by the ancients, they thought it looked like

The Blood Supply to the Heart

The right and left coronary arteries arise from the beginning of the aortic arch. These two arteries then branch into smaller vessels that supply oxygenated blood to the muscles of the heart.

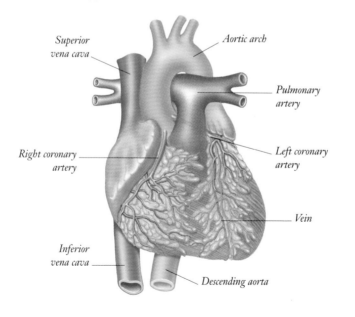

Superior vena cava

Aortic arch

Pulmonary artery

Right coronary artery

Left coronary artery

Vein

Inferior vena cava

Descending aorta

a crown and, in their description, employed the Latin root of the name we use today, the coronary arteries.

Since these arteries are so important, doctors are familiar with all their branches and the variations that can arise from one person to another. The left coronary artery has two main branches, called the anterior descending and the circumflex, which in turn have other branches of their own. The left coronary artery supplies most of the left ventricle, which is the more muscular of the two ventricles because it pumps blood around the entire body. The right coronary artery is usually smaller. It supplies both the right ventricle, which is the chamber that pumps blood to the lungs, and the underside of the left ventricle.

The coronary arteries are similar in structure to all other arteries, but they are different in one way: blood can flow through these vessels into the heart muscle only between beats as it relaxes. While the heart muscle is contracting, the pressure is too great to allow blood to pass through the heart muscle itself. Therefore, the heart requires a very efficient network of fine blood vessels in the heart muscle to get the blood where it is needed.

In CAD, the coronary arteries become narrowed, and the heart muscle becomes starved of needed blood and oxygen. If you are resting, this may not matter. However, if you climb stairs, your heart works harder than normal and needs more oxygen. The coronary arteries may not be able to keep up with this increased oxygen demand, and you get pain in your chest called angina (see pp.39–40). The pain will usually go away if you rest for a while. If a coronary artery becomes completely blocked by a blood clot, the area of heart muscle served by that artery may be permanently damaged, a condition called myocardial infarction (see pp.22–24).

ATHEROMA

Hardening of the arteries, atherosclerosis, and atheroma are all basically the same thing. When you are born, your blood vessels are flexible and elastic, and the blood can flow through them with ease. Early in adult life, however, fat deposits can start to form on the walls of the arteries. They gradually build up, forming lumps that protrude into the inside of the arteries and reduce the blood flow.

The extent of these changes and the rate at which they occur are affected by the level of fats (technically called lipids) in the blood, especially one called low-density lipoprotein (LDL) cholesterol, sometimes referred to as "bad cholesterol" (see p.82). People who have high blood levels of LDL cholesterol are more likely to develop severe atheroma, but some changes may be present in all of us by the time we reach middle age. Those with low levels of high-density lipoprotein (HDL) are also at increased risk.

As the areas of atheroma grow, they thicken and weaken the wall of the artery and progressively reduce blood flow to any organ, affecting its ability to function. Atheroma of the arteries to the brain can lead to a stroke; to the limbs, gangrene; and in the heart, a heart attack.

The process of hardening of the arteries is curiously patchy throughout the body and is particularly so in the coronary arteries. The narrowing can affect just one coronary artery or part of one, or it can affect the artery throughout its length. This may be important in deciding what treatment is best.

In CAD, doctors often talk of one-, two-, or three-vessel disease; this refers to whether the three main branches, the right coronary artery and the two main branches of the left coronary artery, are affected. In general, one- or two-vessel disease may be treated with medication or angioplasty, whereas three-vessel disease, which affects all the major coronary arteries, often requires bypass surgery.

THROMBOSIS

Thrombosis is the medical term for clotting, the natural process that stops bleeding when we injure ourselves. When a blood vessel is damaged, a whole series of chemicals is released at the site of the injury, activating the blood and causing it to clot. In the case of coronary disease, a clot forms, not because of an outside injury but as a result of damage to the lining of the artery caused by the fat that has built up in its wall.

Normally, the lining of our arteries is smooth and does not provide any focus on which a clot can form. When atheroma develops, the lining is no longer smooth. Where there are breaks in the surface of the lining, small cells from the blood called platelets stick to these breaks and help seal them. If the breaks are small, no harm results. However, if the artery is critically narrowed, even a small clot can have an important effect on blood flow. We now know that such a process is the cause of sudden deterioration in unstable angina (see p.40).

In a heart attack, a different process is probably responsible. The fatty deposit in the artery not only contains fat but is also surrounded by scar tissue caused by the cholesterol itself. The scar tissue forms a fibrous cap over the top of the deposit that is much more rigid than the rest of the artery. Any sudden stress can cause this cap to split, creating a wider area

How Does Thrombosis Occur?

The process of thrombosis (blood clot formation) may be triggered by damage to the thickened lining of a blood vessel. The resulting clot may then obstruct the flow of blood through the vessel.

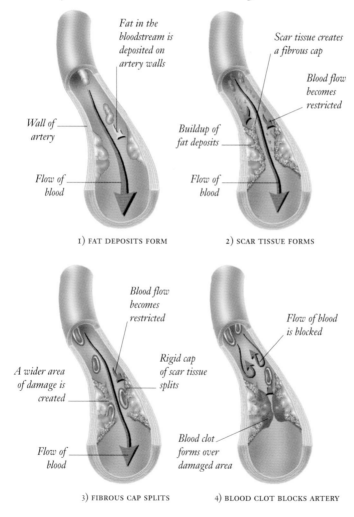

Fat in the bloodstream is deposited on artery walls

Wall of artery

Flow of blood

1) FAT DEPOSITS FORM

Scar tissue creates a fibrous cap

Blood flow becomes restricted

Buildup of fat deposits

Flow of blood

2) SCAR TISSUE FORMS

Blood flow becomes restricted

A wider area of damage is created

Rigid cap of scar tissue splits

Flow of blood

3) FIBROUS CAP SPLITS

Flow of blood is blocked

Blood clot forms over damaged area

4) BLOOD CLOT BLOCKS ARTERY

of damage to the wall of the artery. This results in formation of a much larger clot, one that usually blocks the artery completely. Blood cannot reach the heart muscle beyond this clot, and that section of muscle dies.

Thrombosis is one of the central problems in coronary artery disease. It is the cause of most cases of sudden deterioration in angina and of most heart attacks. The newer and highly effective treatments of coronary artery disease work by removing these clots and preventing their recurrence. Complex and expensive drugs can dissolve a clot in a heart attack and simple, equally effective drugs such as aspirin can prevent them from forming in the first place.

Research is being done to determine what factors make blood clots more likely to form in some people than others.

HEART ATTACK

A heart attack is the final result when the diseased coronary artery becomes completely blocked by a clot or thrombus. The heart muscle, or myocardium, beyond the clot is suddenly starved of blood and oxygen and causes pain. The pain becomes more intense as the minutes pass. Unless the clot disperses by itself, which does not often happen, this area of heart muscle dies within 5–10 minutes, resulting in a heart attack, technically known as a myocardial infarction (MI).

The actual size of the heart attack and the amount of damaged muscle depend on a number of factors. The first factor is the size of the artery; the bigger the artery that is blocked, the bigger the area of damage. The second is that the area of damage is generally greater when other coronary arteries are also diseased.

What Happens in a Heart Attack

In a heart attack, one of the coronary arteries suddenly becomes blocked by a blood clot, cutting off the vital blood supply to an area of the heart muscle.

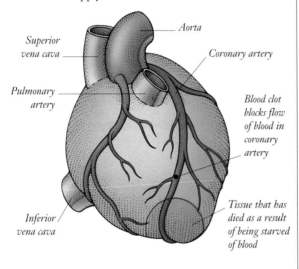

- Aorta
- Superior vena cava
- Coronary artery
- Pulmonary artery
- Blood clot blocks flow of blood in coronary artery
- Inferior vena cava
- Tissue that has died as a result of being starved of blood

Finally, the size of the heart attack depends on whether the area of muscle has developed a collateral blood supply (see p.25). If collateral arteries have developed to supply the threatened area, the damage is much less. Regular exercise is a good stimulus to the formation of collateral vessels, which is one reason why exercise forms such an important part of treatment programs for people with CAD.

The immediate effect of the damage to the muscle, apart from pain, is that the heart no longer pumps as effectively. The blood pressure may fall, leading to faintness and sweating or nausea. The other major problem in the early stages is that the injury to the muscle causes irregularities of heart rhythm, or cardiac arrhythmias. The irregularities can be life-threatening and lead to a condition called cardiac arrest. As a result of the dangers of these arrhythmias, the heart should be monitored closely in the first 48 hours after a heart attack, usually in a hospital cardiac care unit, or CCU. Fortunately, such complications are rare after the first 2–3 days, and most people can return to a general patient unit to recover before going home.

Right after a heart attack, the body begins to repair the damage. Cells remove dead or damaged muscle, and fibrous or scar tissue is formed, a process that takes about 6–8 weeks. The scar itself is strong, but the heart muscle that has been lost cannot be replaced. Some weakening of the heart is inevitable. For most people with a small heart attack, this weakening makes very little difference in the overall performance of the heart as a pump. However, if a larger area of muscle is damaged, the heart becomes enlarged and can no longer pump effectively, a condition we call heart failure.

THE END RESULT

Heart failure can be caused by many diseases affecting the heart, especially high blood pressure. In western countries, however, CAD is probably the most common cause. When the heart stops pumping properly, the lungs become congested with blood, leading to shortness of breath. Congestion in the rest of the body also leads to fluid retention, which causes the ankles and legs to swell. For many years the mainstay of treatment has been the drugs called diuretics, or "water pills," which eliminate the excess fluid in the body and lungs. Now, however, we have a new class of drug called the ACE (angiotensin-converting enzyme) inhibitors, which are even more effective, especially in improving the efficiency of the heart.

The other result of the scarring of heart muscle is that it can interfere with the electrical processes responsible for maintaining the normal heart rhythm and lead to irregularities, or cardiac arrhythmias. The most common irregularity is called atrial fibrillation, which may be treated with digoxin, a drug derived from foxglove. Other irregularities can be treated with drugs such as beta blockers, which are some of the most useful drugs in the treatment of CAD, and newer medications.

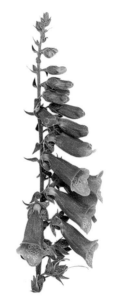

COMMON FOXGLOVE
Digoxin, a well-established drug that is derived from the foxglove flower, is often used to treat atrial fibrillation.

THE EFFECTS OF AGING

Coronary artery disease is a gradual and unpredictable condition. The fatty deposits in the arteries may build up very slowly over the course of 20–30 years. For most of this time, there are no symptoms. Angina becomes a problem only when one or more of the coronary arteries narrow by more than 70 percent and blood flow to that part of the heart muscle is affected.

The process is so slow that the heart can find ways of overcoming the changes by developing new blood vessels called collaterals. The coronary arteries thus form a network of blood vessels around the heart, and, when one is narrowed, one of the other branches expands to help the area of heart muscle affected.

Although the buildup of coronary atheroma is slow, a clot can occur at any time. People who experience only occasional angina may get a sudden worsening of their condition, known as unstable angina, or they may develop a heart attack. Fortunately, unstable angina does not occur very often; annually, only about five percent of people with angina experience such a deterioration.

What is much more worrisome is the fact that a heart attack can occur "out of the blue" in someone who has never been aware of having a heart condition. This can happen because a relatively small fatty deposit, one that causes no real problem in terms of blood flow, can suddenly split. The clot that forms as a result can block off the artery.

We are now beginning to understand this process further. There are a number of drugs that seem to prevent the process.

KEY POINTS

- To function as a pump, the heart muscle depends on the coronary arteries for a good blood supply.
- In CAD, the coronary arteries become narrowed by fatty deposits, or atheroma.
- Narrowing of the coronary arteries can starve the heart muscle of oxygen, resulting in the pain of angina.
- A heart attack results when a diseased coronary artery is completely blocked by a clot. The heart muscle beyond the artery dies.
- After a heart attack, the damaged muscle heals by forming a scar. If the attack is not too extensive, complete recovery can be expected.

Causes of coronary artery disease

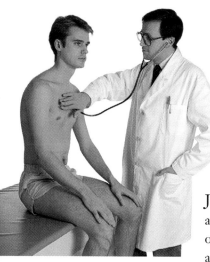

Either there does not exist one single cause of coronary artery disease or we have not yet found it. Medical research has, however, shown that a whole range of risk factors can make you more likely to develop CAD.

CONSULTING YOUR DOCTOR
Regular checkups are advisable if heart disease runs in your family, but there is also much you can do to reduce the risk.

RISK FACTORS

Just as a tall person is more likely to hit his head on a door frame than a shorter one, people with one or more risk factors are more likely to have a heart attack than those without any. Not every tall person hits his head, and, similarly, not every person with risk factors gets a heart attack, but the likelihood is greater.

The risk factors for heart disease are divided into the modifiable, which are those we can do something about, and the unmodifiable, which we cannot change (see opposite). The more risk factors we have, the greater the risk of developing CAD. Not all risk factors are equal. Some, such as smoking, can have a much greater effect on your chances of developing CAD. For example, a smoker with a high cholesterol level and high blood pressure has a much higher risk of heart disease than with just one of these factors.

A high cholesterol level by itself in someone who has no other risk factors increases the risk of heart disease to only slightly above average. This may be nothing to worry about; your doctor will be able to give you individualized advice.

AGE AND GENDER

Heart disease, like many other diseases, becomes more common as people age. In the US, half of the heart attacks occur

Factors that Contribute to the Risk of Developing CAD

MODIFIABLE	UNMODIFIABLE
• Smoking	• Genetic factors,
• High cholesterol	such as an inherited
• High blood	high cholesterol
pressure	level
• Diabetes	• Gender: more men
• Obesity	than women get
• Stress	CAD
• Lack of exercise	• Age

Risk Factors that Affect CAD

Several factors have been found to influence an individual's risk of developing coronary artery disease. The greater the number of risk factors that apply to you, the greater your chance of developing CAD.

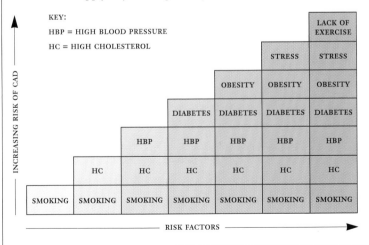

KEY:
HBP = HIGH BLOOD PRESSURE
HC = HIGH CHOLESTEROL

INCREASING RISK OF CAD

					LACK OF EXERCISE
				STRESS	STRESS
			OBESITY	OBESITY	OBESITY
		DIABETES	DIABETES	DIABETES	DIABETES
	HBP	HBP	HBP	HBP	HBP
HC	HC	HC	HC	HC	HC
SMOKING	SMOKING	SMOKING	SMOKING	SMOKING	SMOKING	SMOKING

RISK FACTORS

in people over the age of 65. As the average age of the population increases, the incidence of heart disease also rises.

In people under the age of 55, CAD is much more common among men than women. Before menopause, the change of life when menstruation stops, women have fewer heart attacks. After menopause, CAD becomes more common, and its incidence in women gradually catches up with that in men. Over the age of 75, the numbers are about equal.

The exact reason why women are protected from CAD until they reach menopause is not fully understood. However, it seems likely that this phenomenon is related to the hormones that disappear once menstruation ceases. Now that so many women are taking hormone replacement therapy (HRT), there is some evidence that the treatment may protect against heart attacks. Many doctors recommend HRT for this reason.

FAMILY HISTORY

Doctors talk about a positive family history when one or more close relatives, such as parents, brothers, sisters, or children, have had CAD. If your father suffered from a heart attack before the age of 60 or your mother before the age of 65, your own risk of developing CAD is increased. Of course, if your parents lived to an age at which heart attacks become common, the family history is not as relevant.

The same also applies to brothers and sisters. However, in very large families, the fact that one member may have a heart attack could be just the result of chance.

How does CAD run in families? Part of the answer lies in the genes inherited from our parents, which may

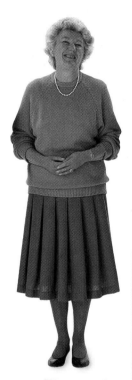

WOMEN AND CAD
Postmenopausal women are just as likely as men to develop CAD. Before menopause, hormones may offer women some form of protection, but the mechanism is not yet fully understood.

make us more liable to have high cholesterol or develop high blood pressure or diabetes. Also, families often live similar lifestyles and eat the same food. Consequently, if the parents smoke, the children often do so as well.

If heart disease appears to run in your family, you should have medical checkups regularly. Make sure that you have not developed high cholesterol, high blood pressure, or other problems that could be treated to reduce your risk.

DIET AND CHOLESTEROL

As we have already seen, atherosclerosis is the major cause of coronary artery disease. Deposits of fat and especially cholesterol, known as plaques, form in the walls of the arteries. This makes the arteries narrower and reduces blood flow. When the plaques split, a clot forms on the damaged area, thereby stopping the flow of blood to a part of the heart muscle. This is what happens in a heart attack. The whole process is more likely to happen and to cause more damage if it does happen in a person who has a high level of cholesterol in the blood.

Your genetic makeup is partly responsible for your cholesterol level. Some families carry genes for elevated levels of various kinds of blood fats. This condition is called familial hyperlipidemia, or FH. Diet also plays an important part in determining cholesterol levels. The more fats you eat, particularly animal and dairy fat, the higher your cholesterol level will be and the higher your risk of CAD (see diagram, p.33). It is important, therefore, to reduce the animal fat content in your diet (see pp.85–86).

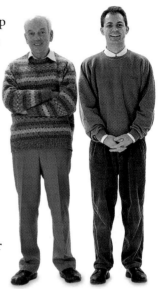

RUNNING IN THE FAMILY
Heart disease may be common in a particular family because of genetic factors or because its members share an unhealthy lifestyle.

THE FRAMINGHAM STUDY

One of the first studies that linked high cholesterol with CAD was carried out after World War II in a small town near Boston called Framingham. All the residents were examined at yearly intervals to see whether they had developed CAD. A strong link with elevated cholesterol was found early in the study; the higher the blood cholesterol, the higher the risk of developing a heart attack. The Framingham Study also showed the importance of other risk factors such as smoking, high blood pressure, and diabetes. These various risk factors have been confirmed over a follow-up period of nearly 40 years since the study first started. The study is ongoing today.

SMOKING AND THE HEART
The more you smoke, the greater the risk of developing heart disease. However, it is never too late to stop smoking. Ex-smokers are less likely to suffer from heart disease than smokers.

SMOKING

Cigarette smoking is strongly linked to the risk of CAD. Chemicals in cigarette smoke are absorbed into your bloodstream from the lungs, circulate around the body, and affect every cell. These chemicals temporarily make the blood vessels narrow. They also cause blood cells called platelets to become stickier, increasing the chance of a clot forming.

Pipe and cigar smokers do not have as high a risk as cigarette smokers but are still more likely than nonsmokers to get CAD. The amount you smoke also matters; the risk rises from light (fewer than 10 cigarettes per day), to moderate (10–20 cigarettes per day), to heavy (more than 20 cigarettes per day).

Doctors stress the importance of stopping smoking because it is a controllable risk. You start to reap the benefits from the moment you stop. Although your risk

Blood Cholesterol Levels

The higher the level of cholesterol in your blood, the greater your risk of developing heart disease. You can lower your risk by changing your diet, particularly by reducing your intake of animal fat.

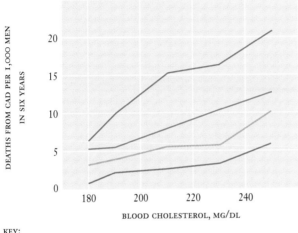

DEATHS FROM CAD PER 1,000 MEN IN SIX YEARS

BLOOD CHOLESTEROL, MG/DL

KEY:

SMOKERS, HYPERTENSIVES

SMOKERS, NONHYPERTENSIVES

NONSMOKERS, HYPERTENSIVES

NONSMOKERS, NONHYPERTENSIVES

of CAD may never be quite as low as that of someone who has never smoked, the risk certainly comes close to that of a nonsmoker a year or so after stopping.

STRESS

Many people who have had a heart attack point to some personal stress as a cause. However, it has been surprisingly difficult to establish this link scientifically. Although there are well-recognized trigger factors, such as sudden unexpected exercise and extreme emotional experiences, that can bring on a heart attack, such factors rarely occur. At times of great civil and military stress, such as in World War II, the number of heart attacks in the civilian population actually fell.

We also tend to think of certain personality types as having a higher risk of heart disease than others. Modern technology has brought with it the ability to do things in an hour that even a generation ago might have taken days. The pressure to take on more than you can manage and set unrealistic goals has created the idea of the type A personality. This restless individual, usually male, finds it difficult to relax and becomes increasingly involved in work at the expense of personal relationships. He is prone to "burnout" and is said to have double the risk of CAD compared with the "laid-back" type B personality.

This theory linking CAD and the stressful personality was once very fashionable, and a lot of effort was devoted to trying to persuade people who had worked hard all their lives to relax. However, modern research has failed to confirm these earlier findings. Although a major illness of any kind is a time to review your priorities, attempts to make major changes in behavior are probably of little benefit.

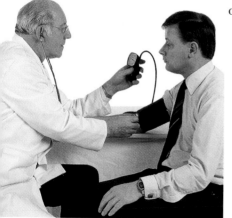

HIGH BLOOD PRESSURE
It is important to have your blood pressure checked regularly. High blood pressure can lead to damage in the arteries, increasing the risk of a heart attack.

▬ DISEASE LINKS TO CAD ▬

Two common and important diseases are associated with a higher-than-average risk of CAD: high blood pressure and diabetes.

- **High blood pressure** The term "blood pressure" actually refers to the pressure in the arteries that take blood from the heart to the rest of the body. High blood pressure causes

The Sequence that Makes Up a Heartbeat

The heartbeat sequence has three phases, diastole, atrial systole, and ventricular systole. The timing of these phases must be accurately maintained, regardless of how slowly or rapidly the heart is beating.

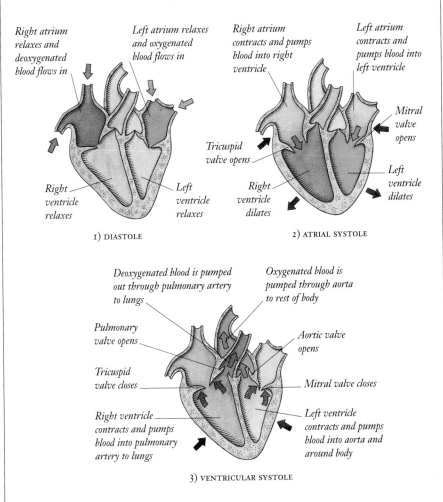

Right atrium relaxes and deoxygenated blood flows in

Left atrium relaxes and oxygenated blood flows in

Right atrium contracts and pumps blood into right ventricle

Left atrium contracts and pumps blood into left ventricle

Mitral valve opens

Tricuspid valve opens

Right ventricle relaxes

Left ventricle relaxes

Right ventricle dilates

Left ventricle dilates

I) DIASTOLE

2) ATRIAL SYSTOLE

Deoxygenated blood is pumped out through pulmonary artery to lungs

Oxygenated blood is pumped through aorta to rest of body

Pulmonary valve opens

Aortic valve opens

Tricuspid valve closes

Mitral valve closes

Right ventricle contracts and pumps blood into pulmonary artery to lungs

Left ventricle contracts and pumps blood into aorta and around body

3) VENTRICULAR SYSTOLE

stress on the heart and circulation. Most people are aware that high blood pressure causes strokes. However, in the US, high blood pressure is responsible for more heart attacks than strokes, probably because of the high cholesterol levels common in this country. Treatment of high blood pressure will reduce the risk of both heart attack and stroke. Blood pressure is usually measured in the upper arm. With each beat of the heart, the blood pressure rises to a high point (systolic pressure), then falls to a low point between beats (diastolic pressure). This pressure is measured in millimeters of mercury (mmHg). An average healthy person's blood pressure at rest is about 120/70, expressed as 120 over 70. A resting pressure of 140/90 is considered borderline, whereas a resting blood pressure of 150/100 is significantly elevated.

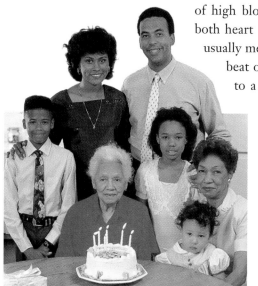

HYPERTENSION
High blood pressure is commonly found among African-Americans.

High blood pressure, known as hypertension, is found around the world and is particularly common in African-Americans. It is also very common in the US as a whole, with perhaps 25 percent of the population over the age of 50 having high blood pressure.

The cause of high blood pressure is not known in most people. It tends to run in families and is seen in people with kidney disease. Unfortunately, in most cases high blood pressure does not cause any symptoms. For this reason, you should have your blood pressure checked from time to time in case it is high and you do not know it.

The high pressure in the arteries damages their lining and accelerates the development of atherosclerosis or atheroma. In addition, high blood pressure forces the heart to work harder at pumping blood to other parts of the body. When atherosclerosis develops in the coronary arteries supplying the heart itself, the supply of oxygen becomes inadequate. This increases a person's chances of developing angina or having a heart attack. High blood pressure also increases the risk of stroke because of the damage caused to blood vessels in the brain.

- **Diabetes** This is a common condition that affects roughly three in 100 people in the US. It is caused by a deficiency of or a resistance to the hormone insulin, which is essential to control the movement of glucose from the bloodstream into cells throughout the body.

Diabetes can affect people of any age, including children. The younger you are, the more likely you are to need insulin injections to control it. Many people get diabetes in middle or old age. When this happens, there are usually few if any symptoms at the time of diagnosis and the condition can most often be controlled by diet and drugs. The aim of treatment is to keep the blood level of glucose as close to normal as possible. However, even with treatment, diabetes can increase the risk of many circulatory disorders, including CAD. It also seems to offset the protective effect of female hormones. Almost as many women as men with diabetes develop CAD.

Good control of diabetes with diet, drugs, or insulin decreases the risk of heart and circulatory problems. Poor diabetes control can often result in very abnormal blood fat levels, including high cholesterol. People with diabetes may need to take additional drugs to control these elevated fat levels.

KEY POINTS

- CAD is more common in men than in women and in the elderly than in the young.
- Important risk factors for CAD are smoking, elevated blood cholesterol, high blood pressure, and diabetes.
- Stopping smoking and reducing cholesterol and blood pressure levels reduce the risk of CAD.

Recognizing the symptoms

Although most people with CAD have the same underlying problem of narrowed coronary arteries, they do not all get the same symptoms. Some develop angina; others may have a heart attack. A smaller proportion of people may develop heart failure without experiencing any warning symptoms. We do not know what determines these outcomes.

CHEST PAIN

Not all chest pain is caused by CAD. You might think that it would be easy to distinguish chest pain caused by heart disease from any other kind of chest pain such as indigestion. However, it can be difficult, even for the most experienced doctor.

- **Angina** "Angina pectoris" is Latin for pain or pressure in the chest. It is brought on by exercise or other stressful activity and goes away when you rest. In CAD, the pain comes from muscle fibers in the heart, which do not have enough oxygen for the work they are doing.

PAIN IN THE CHEST
Pain due to CAD is a dull, crushing feeling that usually starts in the center of the chest and may spread to the neck, arms, and back.

39

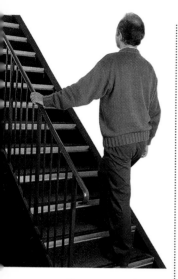

EXERTION AND ANGINA
Climbing a flight of stairs may be enough exercise to bring on the pain of angina.

Angina usually lasts for about 2–3 minutes and no more than 10. It may come on only when you walk uphill or into a strong wind or when you are climbing stairs. However, angina also can come on after mild exertion, such as getting dressed. It is usually worse in cold weather and when you exercise after a meal.

● **Unstable angina** In general, angina is fairly predictable. However, if the coronary artery narrows still further or a clot forms on its surface, the disease can enter a new phase called unstable angina. You may suddenly find that you can only walk a short distance before developing pain, or you may develop pain when you do light work around the house or even when you go upstairs to bed. Sometimes you may be awakened from sleep by an attack of angina. A change in the pattern of pain is an important development and should be reported to your doctor. Unstable angina can lead to a heart attack, and it is important to take preventive steps.

● **Heart attack** The pain of a heart attack is the same as angina but, instead of easing off when you rest, it gets worse. People who have experienced a heart attack often say it is the worst pain they have ever felt in their lives. During a heart attack, they look gray and sweaty and feel cold to the touch. They often feel nauseous and may vomit. Some people who have heart attacks have never had any symptoms of heart disease, and the attack comes out of the blue. However, most people will have had some pain off and on for weeks or months as the blood vessels have gradually become narrower.

How to Recognize Heart Pain

- A dull pain or pressure that does not feel worse when you inhale.
- Usually in the middle of the chest but may spread to the left side, to both arms, or up into the neck or jaw.
- Often described as heavy, burning, vicelike, or like a weight on the chest.

The Stages of Coronary Artery Disease

In a normal heart, the coronary arteries remain clear, providing the heart with adequate oxygen. A narrowed coronary artery will cause angina. When the coronary artery is blocked, a heart attack can result.

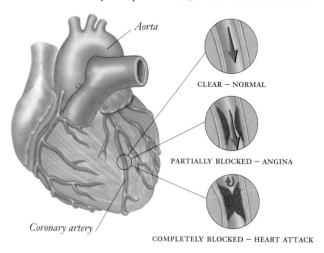

Aorta

CLEAR — NORMAL

PARTIALLY BLOCKED — ANGINA

Coronary artery

COMPLETELY BLOCKED — HEART ATTACK

The difference between angina and a heart attack is that angina leaves the heart muscle short of oxygen but basically undamaged, whereas a heart attack kills part of the heart muscle as a result of oxygen shortage.

In about 20 percent of cases, the symptoms of a heart attack may be mild and are often mistaken for indigestion. This is particularly true in elderly people and those with diabetes, perhaps because the pain fibers to the heart are not as sensitive in these two groups of people.

OTHER CAUSES OF CHEST PAIN

We all experience various chest pains at one time or another. Likely causes include the following:

INDIGESTION OR "HEARTBURN"

The esophagus, or food pipe, which leads from the mouth to the stomach, lies just behind the heart and has the same nerve supply. It is not surprising that pain from the esophagus, commonly called heartburn, may feel much like pain from the heart. Heartburn can occur at any time but is usually related to eating, starting half an hour or so after meals or when the stomach is empty. Indigestion can also occur at night when you lie flat because some of the acid from the stomach spills back into the esophagus and irritates it. Usually, eating more food, drinking milk, or taking antacids eases heartburn. Hot fluids, caffeinated beverages, aspirin and nonsteroidal anti-inflammatory drugs, and alcohol make heartburn worse.

Heartburn is not brought on by exercise. If you feel a pain in your chest when you walk, even if it makes you belch, the pain is much more likely to be from your heart than from your stomach, and you should see your doctor.

PLEURISY

Chest infections such as pneumonia, especially those involving the membrane that covers the lungs, can give rise to chest pain called pleurisy. The pain is usually sharp, only on one side of the chest, and is worse when you cough or take a deep breath. This is different from the dull constant pain from the heart, which spreads across the chest.

MUSCLE PAIN

Along the back and between the ribs, there are muscles that play an important part in breathing and, like all muscles, can be subject to inflammatory pain. This pain is usually confined to a fairly small area of the chest,

Other Types of Chest Pain

Chest pain can be alarming and often causes people to think that they may be having a heart attack. However, there are many other, less serious causes of chest pain, including back injury and infection.

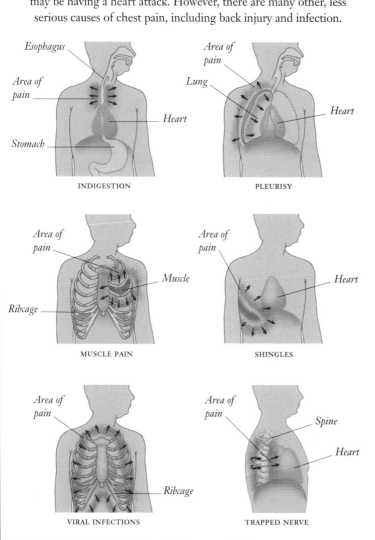

Esophagus

Area of pain

Stomach

Heart

INDIGESTION

Area of pain

Lung

Heart

PLEURISY

Area of pain

Muscle

Ribcage

MUSCLE PAIN

Area of pain

Heart

SHINGLES

Area of pain

Ribcage

VIRAL INFECTIONS

Area of pain

Spine

Heart

TRAPPED NERVE

either at the front or back. It is worse when sitting or lying in certain positions or when you turn around. The pain can last from a few hours to a few days and then may disappear before returning again a few weeks later.

There are other possible causes of chest pain, although they are less common:

- **Shingles** This infection can cause severe pain around the chest for 2–3 days before the telltale blistering rash appears in the painful area.
- **Viral infections** A cold or flulike virus can affect the cartilage that attaches the ribs to the breastbone. When this happens, the chest feels tender when pressed.
- **Trapped nerve** Sometimes, pressure on a nerve in the back or neck can cause pain that spreads down the arm or around the chest. This can be caused by damage to a disk or by arthritis in the spine. Another relatively common cause, especially in women, is collapse of a bone in the spine. This is usually the result of osteoporosis, in which the bones become thin and fragile.

PALPITATIONS

Palpitations, when the heart beats rapidly, irregularly, or misses a beat, are very common in healthy people. They are usually brought on by stress, smoking, or drinking too much coffee or tea. A few people may also have an electrical "short circuit" in the heart that gives rise to a very rapid heartbeat, but this is uncommon.

People with CAD can also develop problems with heart rhythm. However, this usually occurs after a heart attack, and your doctor will then give special drugs to treat the abnormal rhythm. If your palpitations are associated with faintness, shortness of breath, or chest pain, you should tell your doctor as soon as possible.

SHORTNESS OF BREATH

There are many possible reasons for shortness of breath, of which the most common are probably chronic bronchitis, emphysema, and asthma. Heart failure also causes shortness of breath and can affect someone who has had a heart attack (see pp.22–24). If the heart is not pumping properly, fluid tends to build up in the tissues and lungs, and the result is shortness of breath. You may then find it difficult to lie flat in bed or may wake up in the night short of breath. You may also develop a cough yielding a little frothy or blood-stained sputum.

When fluid builds up in your body, you may find that your ankles swell or that you get pain in the stomach because your liver becomes swollen. If you have a heart condition, shortness of breath or a cough that does not go away may be important. There are now effective drugs for treating heart failure, and the sooner you seek help, the better.

KEY POINTS

- The chest pain known as angina or a heart attack can result if the heart muscle is short of oxygen.
- Severe chest pain is assumed to be a heart attack until proved otherwise.
- Angina usually comes on when you exercise or are under stress.
- Indigestion is not usually brought on by exercise; if in doubt, seek advice.

Tests for coronary artery disease

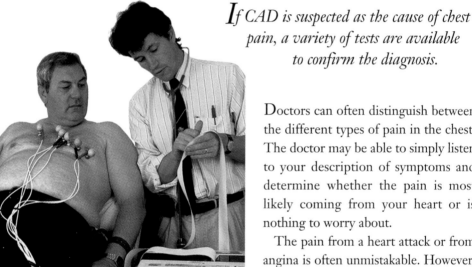

If CAD is suspected as the cause of chest pain, a variety of tests are available to confirm the diagnosis.

HAVING AN ECG
An electrocardiogram helps the doctor investigate and diagnose a wide range of heart diseases. This simple test takes about 5 minutes.

Doctors can often distinguish between the different types of pain in the chest. The doctor may be able to simply listen to your description of symptoms and determine whether the pain is most likely coming from your heart or is nothing to worry about.

The pain from a heart attack or from angina is often unmistakable. However, there are times when the diagnosis is less clear-cut, and the doctor then has to make a decision based upon how likely it is that you have CAD. In a young woman without risk factors for CAD, chest pain is much more likely to be indigestion than angina. In a middle-aged man who smokes and has high blood pressure, it is more likely to be angina than indigestion.

In diagnosing CAD, experience counts, although no doctor is infallible. In actual fact, some doctors have been unable to diagnose their own heart attacks.

Since CAD is so common in the US, most doctors will arrange for further tests if there is any doubt about the diagnosis.

ELECTROCARDIOGRAM

If heart disease is suspected, you will probably have a heart tracing, known as an electrocardiogram. This test will record abnormalities in the electrical pathways of the heart.

RESTING ECG

The most common test that is used for the diagnosis of heart conditions is the electrocardiogram, also known as an ECG or EKG. It is a simple, painless test that takes about 5 minutes and can be conducted by your doctor or nurse.

Every time the heart beats, it causes natural electrical changes that can be picked up by electrodes placed at various points on the body. These electrodes, which are covered in a sticky gel to ensure good contact, are usually put on the ankles and wrists and across the chest.

The ECG records the heart rate and rhythm and shows whether the muscle is conducting electricity normally. Damaged muscle or muscle that is short of oxygen will produce a different tracing.

The ECG gives the doctor a lot of information about the heart, but, like most tests, it is not infallible. Comparing the test to one that you have taken previously may highlight a problem area.

If you have angina, your ECG may still be normal if it is recorded when you are at rest and free of pain. In this case, you may need an exercise ECG.

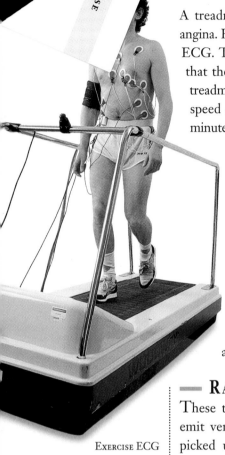

EXERCISE ECG

A treadmill (or bicycle) test can be used to provoke angina. ECG electrodes are attached just as for the resting ECG. The wires are carefully attached to the chest so that they do not come loose while you exercise. The treadmill is usually started at a slow speed, and then the speed and degree of incline are increased every 2–3 minutes. The test is stopped if you develop pain, if there are major ECG changes, or if you become tired or too short of breath.

The useful thing about the exercise ECG is that it gives two pieces of information to the doctor. First, if the test produces pain and ECG changes, it confirms the diagnosis of angina. Second, if you do well and manage to walk a fair distance before the pain comes on, it tells the doctor that the angina is mild and that further tests may not be necessary. The test is usually done in a clinic or hospital and takes about 20–30 minutes.

EXERCISE ECG
Your doctor may perform this test to check the health of your heart. As you walk on a treadmill, your heart rate and the electrical activity of your heart are recorded by electrodes.

RADIOACTIVE ISOTOPE TESTS

These tests make use of chemicals, or isotopes, that emit very small amounts of radioactivity that can be picked up by a special camera. Different tissues in the body take up different isotopes. For the heart, the isotopes used most frequently are thallium and technetium. Both of these are taken up by heart muscle with a normal blood supply but not by muscle that has a poor blood supply. Where there is a narrowing or blockage of a coronary artery, that area of heart muscle will not be seen as well as the rest of the heart. Isotopes are radioactive, but the amount of radioactivity given in these tests is small and equivalent to that used in most standard X-ray procedures. The isotope breaks down quickly, is mostly excreted in the urine, and does not pose any danger to you or anybody else.

The isotope scan is carried out in two stages, once when the heart is stressed and again when it is at rest. The two images are compared. The stress pictures are usually taken after a treadmill test, but, for those who cannot exercise, the effects of exercise may be simulated by drugs, the two most common being dipyridamole or dobutamine, which is given by injection. At the end of the exercise test or after the drug is administered, an injection of isotope is given. You then lie under the camera for about 10–15 minutes while the pictures are taken.

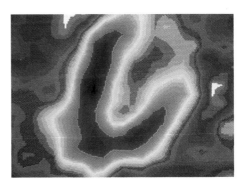

ISOTOPE SCAN

In this colored isotope scan of a normal human heart, the muscle around the left ventricle is seen as a blue/green arc. Areas of heart muscle with reduced blood supply can be detected by this method.

The isotope scan is often better at picking up abnormalities than the exercise ECG and is useful after bypass surgery, when the arterial supply to the heart can be very complicated. The scan is the only way to study the heart in people who cannot manage the treadmill or bicycle because of conditions such as arthritis or lung disease.

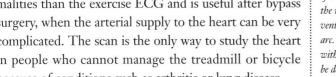

STRESS ECHOCARDIOGRAPHY

This technique is similar in principle to the isotope test except that radioactivity is not involved. The scanner that uses sound beams to take pictures of the heart is called an echocardiogram, and it is just the same as the ultrasound scanner used to see the baby in a mother's womb. With this type of scanner, it is possible to see the heart muscle contracting and also to pick out any

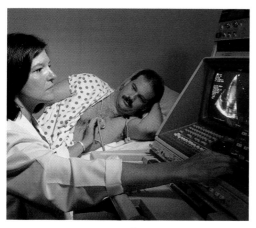

parts that are contracting poorly because the blood supply has been cut off. As in the isotope test, the heart can be stimulated either by exercise or by the injection of drugs such as dobutamine. The heart is scanned before, during, and after the stress. The pictures are then analyzed in detail and can provide good information about which arteries may be blocked and how badly.

CORONARY ANGIOGRAPHY

The most direct way of finding out what is wrong with the heart is to undertake special X-rays of the coronary arteries, called angiograms. In this method, dye that can be seen on an X-ray is injected directly into the coronary arteries. Since the heart is constantly moving, the X-rays have to be taken on film or video, which requires expensive equipment that at one time was available only in a few large teaching hospitals. With modern technology, however, these facilities are now widely available.

In order to take a picture of the heart's small arteries, dye needs to be injected directly into them. To do this, a fine tube called a catheter has to be passed to the heart, usually from an artery in the groin, but sometimes from an artery at the wrist or elbow. A little local anesthetic is injected under the skin to numb the area. The catheter is then passed up through the artery toward the heart. You will not be aware of this happening, although when the tube reaches the heart you may have a few palpitations. This is quite normal. Once the tube is in the coronary artery, dye is injected and pictures are taken from various angles. While this is being done, you will be asked to hold your breath for perhaps 5–10 seconds. The dye itself may cause a little flushing, which passes quickly.

Coronary angiography is a safe and routine procedure. Serious complications rarely occur, less than once in 1,000 procedures. The most important risk, which fortunately is very rare, is that the investigation can provoke a heart attack. If this should happen, emergency surgery may be necessary. Less serious complications include an allergy to the dye or damage to the artery in the groin or the arm. Although coronary angiography is the best way to look at the coronary arteries, it is not necessary for everyone with angina or CAD. Most doctors use it only when there is a real possibility that you might benefit from heart surgery or angioplasty (see pp.58–64).

Coronary angiography is often done as an outpatient procedure and takes about 40 minutes. You probably will not have to stay in the hospital overnight but will need to rest for 4–6 hours after the procedure to reduce the risk of bleeding. The injection site used for the test will often be bruised and may be a little tender for a few days.

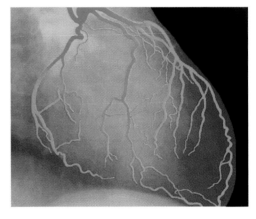

ANGIOGRAM OF THE HEART
This X-ray of the heart, taken after injecting the coronary arteries with a dye, gives a clear view of the arteries that supply the heart.

Key Points

- The most common test for coronary artery disease is the ECG, but it often does not provide enough information.
- If the resting ECG is normal, an exercise test is a good way to show if angina is present and to determine how serious it is.
- For anyone who cannot exercise, pharmacologic radioactive isotope testing or echocardiography can be used instead.
- Coronary angiography is the best way of identifying which arteries are affected, but it is not needed by everyone with CAD.

Treating angina

Angina is pain in the chest caused by inadequate amounts of oxygen reaching the heart muscle. It usually comes on with exercise and disappears after a few minutes of rest. In unstable angina, the condition rapidly gets worse; eventually you are in pain even when resting.

Unstable angina may be a warning of an impending heart attack.

The doctor's aim when he or she is treating angina is to increase the amount of activity or exercise you can do before pain starts and/or to relieve the pain once it has started. Another important goal of treatment is attempting to prevent a heart attack or sudden death in patients with angina. Treatment may be with drugs, angioplasty, or surgery.

TAKING ADVICE
It is important to follow any lifestyle changes that your doctor may suggest, including starting exercise or stopping smoking.

MEDICAL TREATMENTS

Drug treatment is often tried first. Medications work by reducing the amount of oxygen that is needed by the heart muscle, or increasing the blood flow to the heart, or both. Whatever treatment you receive, you should work in partnership with your doctor. Take

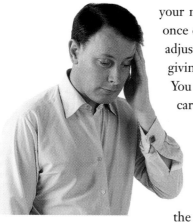

COMMON SIDE EFFECTS
One of the most common side effects of nitroglycerin is a headache, which may occur as the pain from angina subsides.

Warning

IF CHEST DISCOMFORT IS NOT GONE AFTER 15 MINUTES (OR 3 DOSES OF NITRO-GLYCERIN, ONE EVERY 5 MINUTES), CALL AN AMBULANCE FOR TRANSPORTATION TO THE EMERGENCY DEPARTMENT OF THE CLOSEST HOSPITAL.

your medication as prescribed, which is likely to be once or twice a day. In addition, make any necessary adjustments to your lifestyle. This might include giving up smoking, losing weight, and exercising. You will find more about lifestyle changes in Taking care of your heart, on pages 80–91.

NITRATES

Nitrates in various forms have been used for angina for more than 100 years and are among the most common drugs used to relieve the pain of angina. Nitroglycerin is absorbed very quickly through the lining of the mouth and is taken as a small pill under the tongue (sublingually) or as a spray. Nitroglycerin opens up, or dilates, the coronary arteries and improves the blood flow to the heart muscle in areas where the coronary arteries are narrowed.

Nitrates also dilate the arteries and veins throughout the body and can produce side effects, particularly dizziness and headache. If you feel dizzy after using nitroglycerin, sit or lie down for a few minutes. The effect will usually wear off. The headache that often occurs after using nitroglycerin is caused by the dilation of blood vessels to the brain. The pain usually develops within a minute or two of taking the nitrate and disappears quickly if you spit the tablet out.

People often find that the pain from angina starts to ease as the headache develops. The effect of nitrates is so predictable in CAD that doctors may use them to determine whether your chest pain is really angina. Pain in the esophagus, which is located near the heart, can also sometimes be eased by nitroglycerin, which can be confusing.

Anyone who has angina should always keep nitro-glycerin pills or spray on hand in case of an unexpected attack of chest pain. However, if you have opened a bottle of tablets but not used any for a while, keep an eye on the expiration date; nitroglycerin pills are not effective once the bottle has been open for more than six weeks. Nitroglycerin works very quickly. If the pain has not disappeared within five minutes of taking the tablets, something more serious may be developing. Your doctor will probably advise you to wait for five minutes and, if there is no improvement, to take another dose. If your pain is not relieved after three doses of

The Effect of Nitrates on the Heart

In cases of angina, when the blood vessels supplying the heart are constricted, nitrates can be taken to dilate the blood vessels and increase the flow of blood to the heart. As more oxygen becomes available, the strain on the heart is reduced.

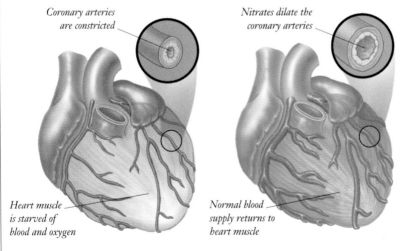

Coronary arteries
are constricted

Nitrates dilate the
coronary arteries

Heart muscle
is starved of
blood and oxygen

Normal blood
supply returns to
heart muscle

DURING AN ANGINA ATTACK

AFTER TAKING NITRATES

55

sublingual nitroglycerin in 15 minutes, call for an ambulance to transport you to the closest emergency department. Time is important, but you should never try to drive yourself.

Nitrates can be swallowed as a pill but are not absorbed well from the stomach. Other, more effective ways of taking them have been developed. Some special formulations include a longer-acting pill called buccal nitrate that can be left between the gum and the cheek for several hours. A skin patch containing nitroglycerin is also available. The transparent patch contains the drug, which is absorbed slowly through the skin. The patch remains in place for 18 hours and is usually removed at night. Your doctor may try several different nitrates to find out which one suits you best.

BETA BLOCKERS

Beta blockers are a group of drugs that were discovered 30 years ago and are a major advance in the treatment of angina. The drugs block the effects of epinephrine on so-called beta receptors in the heart, lungs, and blood vessels. Their effect is to slow down the heartbeat and reduce the blood pressure, particularly during exercise, enabling the heart to do more work before angina develops. Beta blockers often allow people with angina to walk farther than they could before treatment and to reduce the use of nitroglycerin. Sometimes, people find that the angina disappears completely.

Unfortunately, beta blockers do not suit everybody. They cannot be given to people with significant obstructive lung disease or asthma because the drugs make breathing even more difficult. Other possible side effects include cold hands and feet, aching in the leg muscles when walking, fatigue, and occasionally erectile dysfunction. However, more than a dozen different beta blockers are currently available and people often find that one is tolerated better than another.

CALCIUM CHANNEL BLOCKERS

Calcium channel blockers slow the rate at which calcium can enter body cells, particularly in the heart muscle and blood vessel walls, and act like nitrates by dilating the coronary arteries and improving the blood flow to the heart muscle. Like beta blockers, calcium channel blockers increase the amount of exercise you can do before getting angina but do not slow the heart rate. Since they act in a different way from other medications, calcium channel blockers can be used with beta blockers or nitrates, or they can be used by themselves. The most common side effect experienced with these drugs, as with nitrates, are headaches and dizziness. Calcium channel blockers can also cause swelling of the ankles and constipation. This group of drugs has been developed over the last 20 years.

ASPIRIN

Aspirin should be taken by everyone with angina, providing that it is well tolerated. Aspirin works by "thinning" the blood so that clots occur less easily. The danger for someone with angina is that a clot will form in a narrowed coronary artery and lead to a heart attack. By reducing the risk of clot formation, aspirin reduces the risk of a heart attack. The amount of aspirin needed to do this is only 81 milligrams a day, or a quarter of an ordinary aspirin pill. Side effects are rare at this dose, although some people, most often those with asthma, are allergic to aspirin. Others find that aspirin gives them indigestion and therefore they may need to try a coated form of aspirin. Newer anti-platelet drugs such as clopidogrel may provide an alter-native for those who cannot take aspirin.

OTHER DRUGS

Other drugs are being developed for the treatment of angina. Your doctor may wish to use a new drug in your case, either because others have not worked or because they have had side effects.

In some situations, your doctor may also try warfarin, a drug that "thins" the blood even more than aspirin does. Like aspirin, warfarin reduces the risk of a heart attack and may also help angina.

INVASIVE TREATMENTS

If the symptoms of angina become difficult to control with medication, surgery is a treatment option with potentially dramatic results. For example, an individual who has had angina for years can, after surgery, once again walk without difficulty. There are now many procedures that can be used to improve blood flow, either by bypassing arteries (coronary artery bypass surgery, or CABG) or by stretching them (coronary angioplasty, or PTCA).

Although both CABG and PTCA work well, neither treatment is a real "cure." They do not get rid of the basic problem, which is the tendency of the coronary arteries to clog. You must still take steps to keep the arteries from deteriorating, through lifestyle changes such as stopping smoking, with medication, or both (see Taking care of your heart, pp.80–91).

ANGIOPLASTY

Angioplasty was first used about 20 years ago and involves stretching narrowed areas of blood vessels to improve blood flow. It is much quicker and easier than CABG but may be less durable in the long term.

In angioplasty, a long, thin balloon connected to a very fine guide wire is passed across the narrowed region of a blood vessel. The balloon is then inflated at high pressure and stretches the artery, often splitting the fatty deposits in its walls. When the balloon is deflated and removed, the artery remains open.

The problem with coronary angioplasty is that, in about one in four people, the narrowing may return within a few weeks or months. Either the artery is not stretched far enough in the first place or inflammation develops and the narrowing comes back. If either happens, a second angioplasty may be needed. Over the last few years, however, the use of coronary stents has created a big advance in angioplasty.

A stent is a fine wire mesh stretched over the balloon. As the balloon is inflated, the stent stretches with the artery, remaining in place and holding the artery open after the balloon is removed. This helps reduce the risk of a recurrence, known as restenosis.

Unfortunately, this exciting new technique is not suitable for everybody. It is best for people with one or two areas of narrowing in large arteries and is not good for those who have many small narrowed areas or narrowing in all three coronary arteries. In these cases, bypass surgery is a better long-term solution.

How the Balloon Angioplasty Procedure Works

Angioplasty involves widening the affected artery by inserting a balloon along a guide wire and then inflating it at the site of the blockage. Sometimes a fine wire mesh stent is used to hold the artery open to help prevent recurrence.

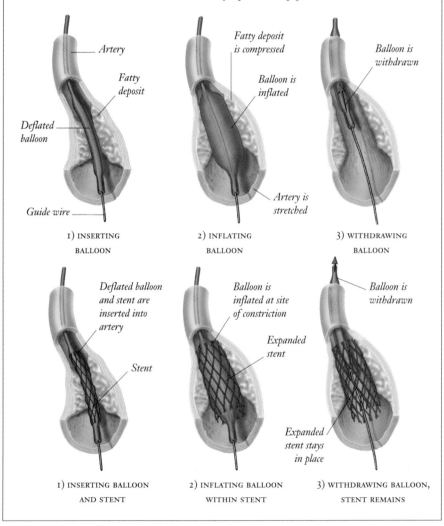

Artery

Fatty deposit

Deflated balloon

Guide wire

1) INSERTING BALLOON

Fatty deposit is compressed

Balloon is inflated

Artery is stretched

2) INFLATING BALLOON

Balloon is withdrawn

3) WITHDRAWING BALLOON

Deflated balloon and stent are inserted into artery

Stent

1) INSERTING BALLOON AND STENT

Balloon is inflated at site of constriction

Expanded stent

2) INFLATING BALLOON WITHIN STENT

Balloon is withdrawn

Expanded stent stays in place

3) WITHDRAWING BALLOON, STENT REMAINS

HAVING AN ANGIOPLASTY

● The procedure is usually done on an overnight basis; you go in one morning and return home the next day. From your point of view, the procedure is similar to having coronary angiography (see pp.50–51).

● A deflated balloon is passed with a fine wire into narrowed areas of the blood vessels and then inflated. The balloon is then removed.

● Some chest pain may occur during the procedure. There is also a 1–2 percent chance that angioplasty may cause a sudden blockage, necessitating emergency bypass surgery. Usually, you will be back to normal after a week.

● Angioplasty can be repeated more than once if it is necessary.

BYPASS SURGERY

Bypass surgery has been one of the major advances in the treatment of angina. The name is derived from the effect of the operation, which is to bypass the blockages in the coronary arteries using replacement blood vessels taken from the chest wall or the legs. You may also hear the term "bypass" used to mean the technique carried out by surgeons when they stop the heart and let the heart–lung machine take over circulation during the operation.

When the operation was first performed, surgeons used veins removed from the legs. These were cut into lengths of 4–5 inches and sewn between the blocked coronary arteries and the aorta, the main artery leading from the heart to the rest of the body.

In the last 10 years the techniques have changed, and if possible, most surgeons now use small artery grafts

Coronary Artery Bypass

Narrow or blocked coronary arteries can be bypassed to restore blood flow to the heart muscle. The bypass may be an internal mammary artery or several vein grafts linking the aorta to the arteries beyond the blockages.

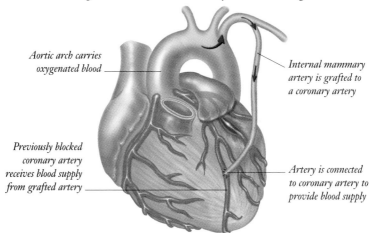

Aortic arch carries oxygenated blood

Internal mammary artery is grafted to a coronary artery

Previously blocked coronary artery receives blood supply from grafted artery

Artery is connected to coronary artery to provide blood supply

MAMMARY ARTERY GRAFTED ONTO THE CORONARY ARTERY

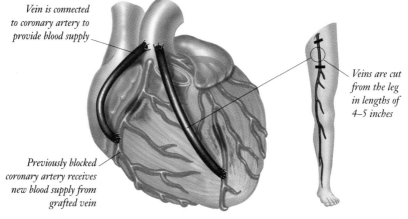

Vein is connected to coronary artery to provide blood supply

Veins are cut from the leg in lengths of 4–5 inches

Previously blocked coronary artery receives new blood supply from grafted vein

VEINS ARE TAKEN FROM THE LEG AND GRAFTED ONTO THE CORONARY ARTERY rather than just vein grafts. The long-term results of this technique appear to be better than they are with veins, which do not withstand the pressures usually present in coronary arteries.

The most commonly used arteries for bypass surgery are the internal mammary arteries, which run down behind the breastbone. These arteries can be attached to either the left or the right coronary artery. More recently, surgeons have even used arteries taken from the stomach or the arm, which may function better than the vein grafts. Commonly, a combination of arterial and vein grafts are used. Of course, major heart surgery is not without risks and is not recommended for everyone with angina, particularly if the symptoms are mild. There are, however, some people with very few symptoms who may need bypass surgery because they have a high risk of a heart attack. Usually, in such cases, angiography has demonstrated that all three coronary arteries are affected (see pp.19–20) or there is significant blockage of the left main coronary artery where it originates at the aorta.

A few people still have angina after CABG because some of the blockages cannot be bypassed. Bypassing all of the main arteries reduces the risk of further heart attacks, but some arteries may be too small for surgery. Residual angina can often be controlled with drugs.

Unfortunately, the new blood vessels may not last forever. If they do become narrowed or blocked, then a second operation or angioplasty may be needed. A second bypass can be more risky than the first. However, the use of mammary arteries may produce long-term results just as good or even better than the conventional techniques.

HAVING A CABG

- You may be admitted to the hospital for 1–2 days before your operation for final tests and assessment. However, more often patients are admitted the morning of surgery.
- On the day of the operation, the anesthesiologist will put you to sleep, and you will wake up after the surgery in an intensive care unit, possibly still on a ventilator.
- You often have a lot of intravenous feedings, drains (tubes in the sacs around the heart and lungs), and monitors for the first 24 hours or so. After that, most of them should be removed. You will then go back to a cardiac recovery area.
- After 4–8 days, you will be able to go home, and, 6–8 weeks later, you should be able to return to most of your normal activities. In other words, you can drive, go back to work except for heavy manual labor, and resume your sex life.

KEY POINTS

- Nitroglycerin taken as a pill or spray under the tongue eases the pain of angina quickly.
- Nitrates, beta blockers, and calcium channel blockers are very effective in controlling angina.
- Aspirin is essential in patients with angina, and it reduces the chances of a myocardial infarction.
- Angioplasty (PTCA) is a technique of stretching the narrowed artery by a high-pressure balloon.
- Coronary bypass surgery (CABG) is very effective in relieving angina and is particularly suitable for advanced disease.

Treating a heart attack

If you have severe pain in the chest and feel cold, sweaty, and nauseated, you are probably having a heart attack. This happens when a coronary artery becomes blocked, usually in an already narrowed artery.

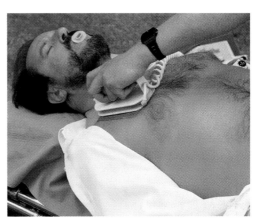

EMERGENCY TREATMENT
A defibrillator is sometimes used to make the heart start beating normally. It works by administering an electric shock to the heart through two metal plates that are placed on the patient's chest.

Ambulance staff, paramedics, doctors, or a combination of all three may treat a person who is having a heart attack. Their aims are the same: to stabilize the heart and reduce the damage done to the muscle.

When medical help arrives, the patient is given oxygen through a face mask, and a plastic cannula, or tube, is inserted into a vein in the arm so that drugs administered enter the bloodstream immediately. ECG leads are attached to the chest to monitor the heart rhythm. The patient may receive morphine for pain.

DISSOLVING THE CLOT

In the early stages after a heart attack, the most important treatment is to restore blood flow, usually with drugs to dissolve the clot or with angioplasty. In some cases, "clot busters" may be started before arrival at the hospital. Although it may sound strange, chewing an aspirin is a good way to start treatment. The aspirin is absorbed through the lining of the mouth and immediately begins to thin the blood.

In addition to aspirin, many new drugs are available. The last 10 years have seen a dramatic change in the treatment of heart attacks because now there are powerful drugs that dissolve the clot blocking the coronary artery. These drugs are administered by injection and are called thrombolytics or, as they are often referred to, "clot busters." Streptokinase is the most common drug used worldwide. In some cases, the more expensive tPA (tissue plasminogen activator) may be preferred.

Thrombolytics work best within the first six hours after a heart attack. After this time, the heart muscle may be too badly damaged even if the artery is unblocked again. Streptokinase is most effective if given in the first hour after a heart attack, but it can still do some good up to 12 hours afterward.

The use of these powerful drugs is not without some risk. However, large trials involving tens of thousands of heart attack patients have shown that the risks are greatly outweighed by the benefits. Since thrombolytics dissolve blood clots, they make people more likely to bleed. In some individuals, this may pose too great a risk. For example, if someone

Treatment Priorities

The priorities of the medical care team in treating a heart attack patient are to:

- Relieve pain and other symptoms, such as nausea.
- Treat any serious cardiac irregularities promptly, with a defibrillator if necessary.
- Restore blood supply to the affected heart muscle by dissolving the clot in the coronary artery.
- Treat complications of the heart attack such as irregular heartbeat or heart failure.

has recently had a major operation, stroke, or bleeding stomach ulcer, other drugs may have to be used.

If streptokinase is administered, you will be given a card to show that you have had it and when.

• This is done because, after five days or so, most people develop resistance to streptokinase. The resistance lasts for a year or more.

• If you need thrombolytic drugs within this period, you will be given the alternative, tPA.

• It is very important that you carry this card with you at all times in case you have to go to a hospital for any reason.

Angioplasty (PTCA) is another way of restoring blood flow to the heart muscle during a heart attack. Not all hospitals perform emergency angioplasty, but, if you are admitted or transferred to a hospital that is equipped to do this, you may receive this treatment instead of clot-dissolving medications. As with the drugs, this technique works best when it is done within the first 4–6 hours after a heart attack. The procedure is similar to routine angioplasty (see pp.58–61), but it carries greater risk because it is being done during a heart attack. Some patients will require angioplasty shortly after being given a clot-dissolving drug if the drug fails to completely dissolve the clot. After a heart attack, many doctors will do angioplasty a day or so later to help improve blood flow to the heart muscle, aiding the healing of the damaged muscle and helping prevent abnormal heart rhythms. Rarely, emergency surgery may be needed if angioplasty does not work or if severe blockages are found in all of the coronary arteries.

══ REGULATING THE HEARTBEAT ══

In the early stages of a heart attack, the damaged heart muscle can become very irritable and produce irregular rhythms, some of which can cause the heart to stop completely. Sadly, this is why when some people develop chest pain, they die before help arrives. These irregularities of heart rhythm, which are known as cardiac arrhythmias, can be treated very successfully by passing a brief electric shock through the heart using a machine called a defibrillator. You may well have seen this treatment depicted on TV or in a movie. People who need defibrillation have always lost consciousness and therefore do not need an anesthetic. Unfortunately, the procedure works only if the shock can be given within a few minutes of the heart stopping, which is why ambulance and paramedic services are so vital. You may also be able to help if you know what to do (see p.91).

In the hospital, people who have had a heart attack are usually treated in a cardiac care unit, where the heart rhythms can be monitored closely for the first 24–48 hours, the danger period. If irregular rhythms start to develop, they can usually be controlled with drug treatment and will not become severe enough to require an electric shock. After this period, the risk of rhythm problems is much lower, and drugs such as beta blockers can be used to prevent recurrence.

══ RECOVERING IN THE HOSPITAL ══

The worst period after a heart attack is the first day or two. During this time, the patient is usually monitored closely. After that, most people have no more pain and are able to get up and around fairly soon. After a straightforward heart attack, some patients may be able to go home in 5–7 days. Others, especially elderly people, may need to stay in the hospital longer.

In the first week, although there is no more pain, patients may feel tired and have a slightly raised temperature, both of which usually clear up as the healing process begins. A scar forms on the damaged area of heart muscle, just as in any other part of the body after an injury. This scarring is more or less complete 4–6 weeks after the heart attack.

People who have never been in the hospital or had anything seriously wrong may need time to come to terms with what has happened. Financial and family commitments may also be a source of concern. Nursing and medical staff are well aware of these problems, and patients should feel free to talk about their concerns. It is time, too, to think about your lifestyle and what you can do to prevent another heart attack (see Taking care of your heart, pp.80–91).

CAUSING CONCERN
The concern that friends and relatives will naturally feel must be kept in perspective. You need to take it easy without being overprotected.

GOING HOME

After all the attention in the hospital, it can feel strange to go home. Patients often worry about what they can and cannot do. A spouse or partner may be even more worried than the patient. It is usually safe to do most things around the house, but, you should avoid all heavy physical activity in the first few weeks. This includes housework, such as vacuum cleaning, which takes more energy than you might think.

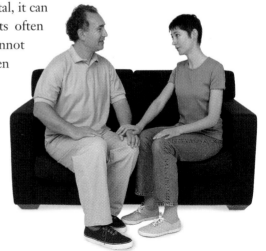

Drugs Your Doctor May Prescribe

After a heart attack your doctor will prescribe drugs to prevent a recurrence.
This chart includes some of the more common drugs, but there are many others.

CLASS OF DRUG	GENERIC NAME*	ADMINISTRATION	PURPOSE	POSSIBLE SIDE EFFECTS
Salicylates	Aspirin	Pills	Thin blood	Gastric upset
Nitrates	Nitroglycerin	Under the tongue, in the cheek; tablets, skin patches, ointment, or spray	Relieve angina	Flushing, headache
	Isosorbide dinitrate	Pills, capsules, or under the tongue		
	Isosorbide mononitrate	Pills		
Beta blockers	Acebutolol	Capsules	Slow heart rate, protect against heart attack	Fatigue, lethargy, cold hands, nightmares, dizziness
	Atenolol	Pills or syrup		
	Bisoprolol	Pills		
	Labetalol	Pills		
	Metoprolol	Pills		
	Nadolol	Pills		
	Pindolol	Pills		
	Propranolol	Pills, capsules, syrup		
	Timolol	Pills		

Drugs Your Doctor May Prescribe (cont'd.)

CLASS OF DRUG	GENERIC NAME*	ADMINISTRATION	PURPOSE	POSSIBLE SIDE EFFECTS
Calcium antagonists	Amlodipine Diltiazem Felodipine Nicardipine Nifedipine Nisoldipine Verapamil	Pills or capsules Pills or capsules Pills Capsules Pills or capsules Pills Pills or capsules	Relieve angina	Flushing, headache, ankle-swelling, constipation
ACE inhibitors	Captopril Enalapril Fosinopril Lisinopril Ramipril Quinapril Trandolapril	Pills Pills Pills Pills Pills or capsules Pills Pills	Protect against heart failure	Persistent dry cough, dizziness, occasional diarrhea
Statins	Atorvastatin Cerivastatin Fluvastatin Pravastatin Simvastatin	Pills Pills Capsules Pills Pills	Reduce cholesterol	Headache, indigestion, occasional muscle inflammation

Pharmaceutical companies give their products brand names. Only the generic names are listed here; you will be able to find the generic name on the package of your medication.

It is very important in these early stages that family and friends try not to be too overprotective.

Even a little twinge of pain may become larger than life. After a heart attack, most people become much more aware of aches and pains that would previously have been ignored. A reported 90 percent of people experience some form of noncardiac pain in the first few weeks after a heart attack. About one in three people experience angina, which may feel similar to a heart attack. Angina usually coincides with effort and eases with rest. In the event of chest pain, take nitroglycerin. If the pain persists after using nitroglycerin, take another dose, and, if necessary, a third dose. If the pain lasts more than 15 minutes, you should call an ambulance for immediate transportation to the closest emergency department. Never attempt to drive yourself.

— TAKING MEDICINES AT HOME —

During the first week in the hospital, you will be given a variety of drugs, some to treat complications and others to reduce the risk of further problems.

A wide variety of drugs are available for people who have had a heart attack. Your doctor will decide which is best for you. Do not be surprised if you know someone who has been given different medication, because drugs must be tailored to suit the needs of each individual.

• **Aspirin** This is the most commonly prescribed drug. Some people cannot take it, usually because of severe stomach problems. Aspirin reduces the stickiness of platelets, the blood cells that are involved in clotting.

• **Beta blockers** These drugs block the effect of epinephrine on receptors in the heart and blood vessels, reducing the risk of another heart attack and cutting the mortality rate. Many physicians routinely prescribe beta blockers after a heart attack. Some people cannot take them because of asthma or obstructive lung disease.

● **ACE inhibitors** These are a major advance in the treatment of heart problems. Angiotensin-converting enzyme, or ACE, increases the blood level of angiotensin. Angiotensin constricts blood vessels and causes the body to retain more salt and water than normal. By reducing angiotensin levels, ACE inhibitors have decreased the occurrence of heart attacks and heart failure.

● **Statins** These are potent new drugs that lower cholesterol. Statins reduce the amount of cholesterol that is made in the body, particularly in the liver, and help prevent further clogging of arteries (see pp.83–84). In this circumstance, they may be prescribed even if your blood cholesterol level is not elevated.

● **Nitroglycerin** You are likely to be prescribed this drug for chest pain, either in a spray or a pill. Use it if you experience chest pain after you leave the hospital; make sure you know how and when to take this drug.

KEY POINTS

- Prompt treatment is vital. Call an ambulance rather than your doctor.
- Close monitoring is required in the first few days, usually in a cardiac care unit (CCU).
- Most people can expect to recover fully from a heart attack in 6–8 weeks.
- Drugs are used to prevent a recurrence.

Recovering from a heart attack

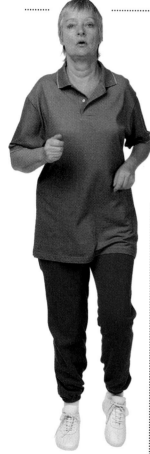

At one time, doctors would have insisted that you stay in bed for 6–8 weeks after a heart attack, in the mistaken belief that this would facilitate healing. It was not surprising that, after such a long period in bed, people felt worse than they did during the attack.

REHABILITATION

Rehabilitation after a heart attack is very different now than it was in the past. The pain and general weakness usually go away in a few days. The emphasis is then on returning to normal over the next 6–8 weeks.

Most hospitals now have a cardiac rehabilitation, or "rehab," service. The aims of cardiac rehabilitation are:

- **Education** Understanding the cause of the problem and how you are going to get better.
- **Exercise** A graded exercise program to help you return to your normal activities.
- **Prevention** The steps you can take to avoid having another heart attack.

The rehabilitation program usually begins in the hospital when a nurse visits you and tries to answer some of the questions that may be troubling you and your family. You should be given some guidance

EXERCISE AND THE HEART
A regular exercise program is extremely important in maintaining a healthy heart.

regarding what you can and cannot do when you leave the hospital.

An exercise program usually starts 2–4 weeks later and is supervised by a physical therapist. There will probably be other people going through the same program, which will give you a good opportunity to talk and share experiences. It is often very reassuring to see someone exercising very energetically as he or she comes to the end of the program, especially when you are just starting and are worried about exercising at all.

For many middle-aged people, this regular exercise may be the first they have done for years and may seem strange at first. However, most people find the exercise becomes easier and easier as the weeks go by. You are likely to feel better at the end of the program than you have in years.

Rehabilitation sessions usually last 1–2 hours and should take place twice a week for 6–8 weeks. Exercise can be accompanied by discussions about the cause of heart attacks and about their prevention. There may also be visits from a pharmacist, dietitian, and cardiologist to answer any questions you or your family may have about your condition.

RETURNING TO NORMAL LIFE

You may be worried about performing your normal activities, such as work or sexual activity, in the first few weeks or months after a heart attack.

DRIVING

You are usually not allowed by law to drive your car for one month after a heart attack. You do not need to notify your state department of motor vehicles, but you should probably tell your insurance company. There are special regulations for people who drive for a living, such as bus drivers and truck drivers, and these should be discussed with a doctor. In some towns, such regulations may apply to taxi drivers as well.

SEXUAL ACTIVITY

After a heart attack, many people worry about having sex. At first, you do not usually feel like having intercourse. However, it is certainly reasonable to start sexual relations again 3–4 weeks after a heart attack. You should avoid being too vigorous until you feel fully recovered, which normally occurs in about 6–8 weeks. Some of the drugs you may be taking can reduce your sex drive. If this is the case, you should discuss it with your doctor.

WORK

Many people can go back to work 1–2 months after a heart attack. For a physically undemanding job that does not involve much exertion, 4–8 weeks off work may be enough. For heavy manual work, a longer recovery time may be necessary. Special exercises to rebuild strength should be included in the program.

VACATIONS

For the first 2–3 months after a heart attack, it is usually unwise to travel, especially to foreign places. Later, after you have made a full recovery, you can probably travel wherever you like. If in doubt, discuss your plans with your doctor. If you do travel, make sure that you are fully insured and that the insurance policy does not exclude people who have a heart condition. If you are on medication, make sure you have enough to last while you are away, and keep the drugs in your hand luggage.

ANXIETY AND DEPRESSION

Everyone worries after a heart attack. Despite all the encouraging advice from doctors, nurses, and relatives, some people worry excessively. You may have some concern about having another heart attack. It is natural to be worried about yourself and your family, even if it is difficult to put into words exactly why. A heart attack can be a blow to your self-confidence, especially if you have never had any serious health problems before. Consequently, it is relatively easy to become depressed.

RECOGNIZING THE PROBLEM

Depression is as real an illness as heart disease and also just as treatable. You may be depressed if you have several of the following symptoms:

- Sadness or tearfulness.
- Loss of enjoyment or interest in work and hobbies.
- Loss of interest in sex.
- Low self-esteem.
- Preoccupation with your health.
- Poor concentration.
- Sleep disturbance, difficulty getting to sleep, or waking early.
- Constant fatigue.

In depression, the levels of chemicals that transmit signals to the brain are altered; treatment with anti-depressants can bring them back to normal. Unlike tranquilizers, these drugs are not addictive. You will be

GOING ON VACATION
Once you have recovered from a heart attack, long trips are possible if you are fully insured and take the necessary medication with you.

able to stop taking them once you have fully recovered from your depression. Antidepressant medication is usually taken for at least 3–6 months.

In the first few weeks after a heart attack, there are so many things going on and so much to think about that depression may not be obvious. However, once things start to get back to normal, you may have more time to worry about the future. This is when problems can occur.

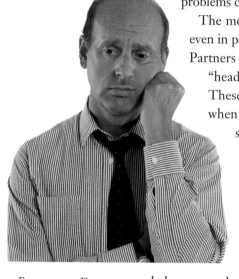

The most common reaction is a short temper, even in people who are generally mild-mannered. Partners often complain that they get their "head bitten off" for the slightest thing. These problems usually settle down if and when the person returns to work and life starts getting back to normal, but some people continue to have a "short fuse" for much longer.

Anxiety and depression are common and can be helped. Often just discussing how you feel with someone else who has been through the same things is all you need. Join a self-help group that gives long-term support if needed. If you have any of the symptoms listed on page 77, do not just wait for them to go away. Consult your doctor.

EXPERIENCING DEPRESSION
If you are suffering from depression, it is important to get help. Talking to others who have had the same experience may be helpful.

KEY POINTS

- Most problems occur in the first 48 hours after a heart attack; after that, life soon returns to normal.
- Regular exercise can help you make a full recovery, but it should be supervised.
- Emotional problems after a heart attack are common and can be helped by talking about them and sometimes with medication.

Taking care of your heart

It is not too late to think about prevention if you have had a heart attack or have developed angina. There are plenty of ways to prevent the heart from deteriorating further. You can reduce your chances of having another heart attack if you reduce your risk factors. Prevention is especially important after bypass surgery because your new blood vessels will be less likely to clog if you take good care of yourself.

REDUCING THE RISKS
Many factors, such as diet, contribute to heart disease. By eating healthily and reducing the amount of fat you eat you reduce the risk of disease.

As we have already seen (pp.28–38), risk factors fall into two distinct categories: those over which you have no control and those that you can influence.

Other diseases, notably diabetes and high blood pressure (hypertension), can increase the risk of developing CAD and are risk factors that fall between the two categories. You may not be able to control the existence of the disease, but the risk is reduced if the conditions are well controlled with the proper medication.

LOWERING CHOLESTEROL

Lipids is the collective term used by doctors to refer to fatlike substances in the blood. Cholesterol is the best-known lipid, but another type called triglycerides may also play a role in CAD.

Cholesterol has a bad reputation as a cause of disease of the heart and blood vessels. However, it also performs some essential functions in the body and no one could do without it entirely. Cholesterol is manufactured in the liver and used in the cell membranes both to make bile and to form vital chemical messengers, or hormones. Therefore, even if you completely excluded cholesterol from your diet, you would always have some in your blood.

Most diets in western countries include large amounts of animal fat that the body converts into cholesterol.

Drugs for High Cholesterol

There are a number of drugs available to bring down the level of fatlike substances, known as lipids, in the blood. Here is a partial list.

DRUG GROUP	GENERIC NAMES	TRADE NAMES
Statins	Simvastatin	Zocor
	Pravastatin	Pravachol
	Fluvastatin	Lescol
	Atorvastatin	Lipitor
	Cerivastatin	Baycol
Fibrates	Gemfibrozil	Lopid
Resins	Colestipol	Colestid
	Cholestyramine	Questran

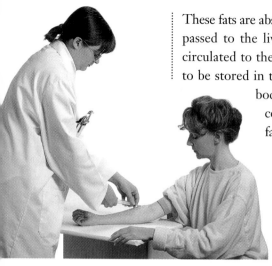

CHOLESTEROL TESTING
A simple blood test can provide an accurate measure of the amount of cholesterol in your blood.

These fats are absorbed by the stomach and intestines and passed to the liver, where they are broken down and circulated to the rest of the body to provide energy or to be stored in the fat cells. Fat circulates through the body in the bloodstream in tiny particles containing mixtures of cholesterol, other fats, and proteins.

When you have a blood cholesterol test, the laboratory usually measures several other fats as well. The total cholesterol level is made up of two parts, which are called low-density lipoprotein (LDL) and high-density lipoprotein (HDL). LDL is the "bad" cholesterol, and, when the level is too high, it builds up in the arterial walls to produce atheroma. About two-thirds of the cholesterol in the blood is LDL, and this is usually what doctors are referring to when they say you have a high cholesterol level.

HDL is, on the other hand, a "good" cholesterol. The higher the level, the less likely you are to get heart disease. Women have higher HDL levels than men do, but this difference usually disappears after menopause.

Triglycerides are the third type of fat that is measured in a blood sample. This type makes up most of the fat in the fat cells of your body and, when released, provides the energy you need for everyday activities. Although triglycerides are not found in any quantity in the fatty deposits in arterial walls, high levels of triglycerides in the blood are indirectly linked to CAD.

Most people who have angina or a heart attack have high lipid levels, which is partly genetic and partly the result of their diet. By careful dieting, we can reduce our lipid or cholesterol levels by 10–20 percent. If we want to lower the levels more than this, drugs are usually necessary. Exercise is helpful in raising levels of "good" HDL cholesterol.

You may find that your doctor prescribes more than one drug to lower lipids because the drugs work in different ways. However, you will also be given advice on reducing the amount of cholesterol in your diet, which is necessary if the drug treatment is to be fully effective (see pp.85–86).

STATINS

The big change in the treatment of cholesterol in the last five years has been the development of statins, a class of drug that functions by slowing the production of cholesterol in the liver. Statins lower cholesterol by 20–30 percent and have very few side effects. They may have a beneficial effect on cardiovascular disease even in those with normal cholesterol levels.

There have now been several important studies showing that this reduction in cholesterol is followed by a 20–30 percent reduction in the risk of further heart attacks. Two of the most common statins currently being used are simvastatin and pravastatin; however, many more are now available.

Statins are usually taken as a single dose with the main meal of the day and have few side effects. Very occasionally, they may cause inflammation in the muscles of the arms and legs, an aching that feels like the flu. This occurs during the first few weeks after starting treatment and should be reported immediately to your doctor. The symptom goes away once the pills are stopped. The drugs may also cause some elevation in the liver enzymes, although this usually causes no symptoms. You will have regularly scheduled blood tests if you are prescribed this type of medication.

If you experience no problems with these drugs in the first few weeks of use, you are unlikely to develop them later.

FIBRATES

For some individuals, particularly those who have diabetes, the problem with the lipids may be not so much with cholesterol as with triglycerides. In that case, another group of drugs called fibrates may be used. Like the statins, these medications have few side effects and are taken with the main meal of the day. They too may produce muscular pains in the first few weeks. In addition to their effect on triglyceride levels, fibrates can reduce cholesterol levels by 10–15 percent and cut the risk of CAD by about the same percentage.

RESINS

Resins reduce cholesterol levels by binding cholesterol in the intestines and thereby affecting the absorption of cholesterol into the body. Resins are taken in the form of a powder, usually in fruit juice, two or more times a day. Since they are not absorbed into the body, they usually do not cause any serious side effects. However, they can cause gas and belching or constipation in some people.

Resins have also been shown to reduce the risk of further heart attacks, but they are less potent than the statins and reduce the risk by only 10–15 percent.

IMPROVING THE DIET

Changing the type of food that you have eaten all your life may not be easy, but it is an important way to reduce the risk of further heart attacks. The basic rules are fairly simple and are given in the box on page 86.

Eating right does not mean giving up everything you enjoy or eating nothing but rabbit food. Most people consume far more fat, especially animal or dairy fat, than is good for them, and cutting down would be a health benefit for the entire family. Red meat, hard cheeses, butter, cream, whole milk and yogurt, and cooking fats such as lard are all high in so-called saturated fats. It is wise to eat relatively less of these foods or just keep them for special occasions.

In addition to reducing the overall amount of fat in your diet, use polyunsaturated fats, generally those from vegetable sources that are liquid at room temperature, or monounsaturated fats, such as olive oil, rather than animal or dairy fat whenever you can. If you are not sure which oils are healthy, check the label or ask a dietitian because there are one or two vegetable oils that are not good for the heart. Coconut oil in particular is nearly almost as bad for the heart as lard.

Cutting down on fats in general is also a good way to lose weight. After changing their diet, many people also suffer much less from indigestion.

You may be concerned about your cholesterol levels and anxious to avoid foods that contain cholesterol, including eggs, organ meats, and shellfish. Although such foods do contain some cholesterol, they are probably

EATING WELL
A high-fiber diet, rich in fruit and vegetables, will benefit your overall health.

Four Steps to Healthy Eating

Anyone can eat well by following these simple guidelines.

- Cut down the total amount of fat in your diet.
- Replace animal fats, including dairy fats, with vegetable oils.
- Eat more fresh fruit and vegetables.
- Go on a sensible weight-reducing diet if necessary.

less significant sources for most people than foods high in animal fats. Bear in mind that many processed and prepared foods such as pies, cakes, and cookies may be high in animal fats, as are more obvious sources such as hamburgers. More health-conscious people take note of the labels on foods in the stores, which give some idea of their fat content.

The other major change that will improve your diet is to eat as much fruit and vegetables as possible, at least five portions every day. If you can also increase your intake of other fiber-rich foods such as brown rice, and whole grain bread, pasta, and breakfast cereals, especially oats, you will be well on the way to a diet that is good for your overall health as well as your heart.

Fortunately, the food industry is beginning to realize the importance of a healthy diet. There are now many excellent cookbooks to help you improve your diet. What many writers ignore, however, is the higher price of some healthy foods. This cost often puts a strain on the family budget. A dietitian may be able to give you advice on the best way to minimize your weekly shopping budget.

STOPPING SMOKING

The benefits of stopping smoking are real and start from the day you quit. Five years later, your risk of having another heart attack will be halved. You have to stop completely, however; just cutting down or changing from cigarettes to cigars or a pipe does little to reduce the risk. Doctors realized this 30 years ago when the research linking heart disease and smoking was first published.

Many people find it easy to stop smoking in the hospital and very hard to keep it up when they go home. If you have smoked since you were a teenager, stopping can be a real problem. Your family can help. If family members smoke, ask them to do so outside. Hospitals are now "no smoking" areas and your home should be, too.

What is the best way to quit smoking? It is different for everyone. Some people find it easiest to stop suddenly. Others prefer to stop gradually, perhaps cutting down by a cigarette a day over several weeks. Part of the problem is an addiction to nicotine itself. For some smokers, the use of nicotine chewing gum or skin patches is a great help. There are also prescription medications that are quite effective in aiding smoking cessation.

Sometimes talking to other smokers who are trying to quit is the best help. Many hospitals and community centers run programs to help people stop smoking. Some people swear by hypnosis.

One of the things that keeps people smoking, especially women, is the tendency to put on weight after quitting. Researchers are still not sure why this happens. Certainly the appetite improves. Some people eat candy to reduce their craving for a cigarette. On average, most people put on 7 to 14 pounds in the first six months after they stop smoking. However, if you change to a healthier, low-fat diet at the same time, the extra weight usually comes off again gradually over the next 6–12 months.

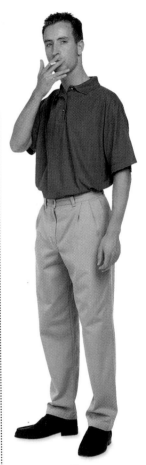

THE SMOKING FACTOR
Smoking greatly increases your risk of suffering from heart disease. However, after you give up smoking, the risk of CAD declines rapidly.

87

REDUCING STRESS

If you develop angina or have had a heart attack, it is an opportunity to evaluate the priorities in your life. You may feel that a job that has occupied a large proportion of your time and energy over the years is now less important to you than family, friends, and other interests. Although there is no scientific proof that changing the way you live reduces your risk, it can certainly improve the quality of your life.

PROTECTIVE FACTORS

Factors that may offer some protection against coronary artery disease include a moderate alcohol intake and regular exercise.

ALCOHOL

There has been a lot of publicity recently about the beneficial effects of alcohol when taken in moderation. However, high levels of alcohol taken regularly can poison the heart, brain, and liver.

What is moderation? The amount of alcohol that seems to be good for you is around 2–3 units a day; women should adhere to the lower end of the range. A unit is an ounce of liquor, a glass of wine, or 11 fluid ounces of beer. Although it was first thought that red wine was particularly effective in preventing heart attacks, it now seems that any form of alcohol has the same effect.

EXERCISE

Regular exercise is also good for you and can protect against CAD. Many studies show that people who exercise regularly (for at least 20 minutes, 3 times a week) have a reduced risk of CAD when compared with the "couch potatoes" of the world.

Recognizing a Unit of Alcohol

Various drinks contain different amounts of alcohol. A unit of alcohol is equivalent to approximately 8–10 grams of pure alcohol.

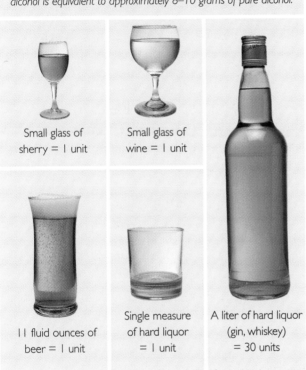

Small glass of sherry = 1 unit

Small glass of wine = 1 unit

11 fluid ounces of beer = 1 unit

Single measure of hard liquor = 1 unit

A liter of hard liquor (gin, whiskey) = 30 units

WHAT IS A UNIT?
Since different drinks contain different amounts of alcohol, alcoholic consumption is measured in units. Recommended intake is 2–3 units a day.

If you have had a heart attack, you will be taught about exercise in your rehabilitation sessions. However, anyone who has any form of CAD may need more exercise. If you have never exercised before and are unsure how to start, ask your doctor for advice. The type of exercise you do is probably not important, providing that it stimulates the heart and circulation sufficiently. Do what you like best. Walking, swimming, jogging, exercising in the gym, and dancing will all help. Most people need to start slowly and gradually build up to longer and more strenuous sessions. If you go to a gym or exercise class, you should be shown how to warm up properly beforehand. It is a good idea to warm up before any exercise session.

The idea of exercising until it hurts and beyond has been thoroughly discredited. If you feel pain or dizziness or find it hard to breathe, stop and rest. You should take a complete break from exercise if you are injured or not feeling well.

WORKING WITH YOUR DOCTOR

Smoking and elevated lipid levels are major risk factors that are largely under your own control. There are other areas in which you and your doctor can work together to minimize the risk of further problems. For example, people with diabetes or high blood pressure (hypertension) need to maintain good control because these conditions increase the risk of CAD (see pp.34–37).

HYPERTENSION

Make a big effort to take your medication regularly, even though you have no symptoms. See your doctor for regular blood pressure measurements.

DIABETES

You should try to keep your weight as close as possible to what it should be for your height. Do your best to keep your blood glucose levels within the normal range by paying careful attention to your diet and by taking the prescribed treatment properly, whether insulin or oral hypoglycemic agents. Exercise to help reduce both your weight and your insulin requirement.

HIGH LIPID LEVELS

Make an effort to stick to your diet and take any medication as prescribed.

⸺ DEALING WITH AN EMERGENCY ⸺

Everyone should know how to help someone whose heart stops beating. Cardiopulmonary resuscitation (CPR) is not difficult and can literally save someone's life. Instruction is available from the American Red Cross, volunteer agencies, or at the local hospital.

If you or someone you are with develops chest pain that seems similar to the heart pain associated with an earlier heart attack, the basic steps to follow are:

- Rest by sitting or lying down.
- Take nitroglycerin and wait five minutes.
- If the pain is still as bad or worse after 5 minutes, take a second dose. Repeat after 5 minutes if necessary.
- If this has no effect, call for an ambulance.
- Chew on an aspirin, unless you know that you are allergic to it. Aspirin will start to thin the blood and discourage clotting.

KEY POINTS

- Changing to a healthy diet improves your fitness.
- Drug treatment to lower cholesterol reduces the risk of CAD.
- Stopping smoking reduces your risk further and is effective immediately.
- Regular exercise benefits your heart and circulation.

Emergency Methods – ABC

In an emergency, it is important to check the ABC functions: Airway, Breathing, and Circulation.

AIRWAY

Make sure that nothing prevents air flow through the nose and mouth.

BREATHING

Check for spontaneous breathing.

CIRCULATION

Feel for a pulse in the neck.

If there is no breathing and no pulse, a cardiac arrest has probably occurred. Call for help. If you have been trained in the technique, begin cardiopulmonary resuscitation immediately.

Useful addresses

American Heart Association
National Center
Online: www.amhrt.org
7272 Grenville Avenue, Dallas, TX 75231
Tel: (800) AHA-USA1
The American Heart Association is a
nationwide public advocacy group that
sponsors public and professional educational
materials, publications, and family health
programs and products.

Salud para su Corazon
Latino Cardiovascular Health Resources
Contact the National Institutes of Health,
below, through their website.
This department of the NIH provides
educational materials in Spanish and English
for the general public and for community
health planners.

NIH National Heart, Lung, and Blood
Institute
Online: www.nhlbi.nih.gov
Building 31, Room 4A-21, 31 Center Drive,
MSC 2470, Bethesda, MD 20982-2470
Tel: (800) 575-WELL
Tel: (301) 251-1222
Like other branches of the National
Institutes of Health, the NHLBI conducts

basic research, clinical investigations and
trials, demonstrations, and educational
projects. Its emphasis is on prevention.

Heart Information Service
Texas Heart Institute
Online: www.tmc.edu/thi
PO Box 20345, MC4-298
Houston, TX 77225-0345
Tel: (800) 292-2221
The Texas Heart Institute, the largest
cardiovascular center in the world, is a
chartered nonprofit institution that provides
health care, research, and medical education.
Their website has links to related sites and
news articles about cardiovascular disease
prevention, treatment, and research.

Heart to Heart Volunteers
Online: www.csusm.edu/public/guests.hhv
PO Box 16
Escondido, CA 92033
Tel: (760) 489-6299
Heart to Heart is an organization of support
groups, educational programs, hospital
visitor programs, with a website and a
nationally distributed newsletter for
patients, families, and doctors of those who
have had "heart events."

Index

Acknowledgments

PUBLISHER'S ACKNOWLEDGMENTS
Dorling Kindersley Publishing would like to thank the following for their help and participation in this project:

Managing Editor Stephanie Jackson; **Managing Art Editor** Nigel Duffield; **Editorial Assistance** Judit Z. Bodnar, Mary Lindsay, Jennifer Quasha, Ashley Ren, Design Revolution; **Design Assistance** Sarah Hall, Marianne Markham, Design Revolution, Chris Walker; **Production** Michelle Thomas; Elizabeth Cherry.

Consultancy Dr. Tony Smith; Dr. Sue Davidson; **Indexing** Indexing Specialists, Hove; **Administration** Christopher Gordon.

Illustrations (p.15, p.17, p.41, p.43, p.55, p.60, p.62) ©Gillian Lee; (p.10, p.21, p.29) Passmore Technical Art Services.

Picture Research Angela Anderson, Andy Samson; **Picture Librarian** Charlotte Oster.

PICTURE CREDITS
The publisher would like to thank the following for their kind permission to reproduce their photographs. Every effort has been made
ıny

7;
ıns),
ix),
p.36.